Praise for
Transforming
Interprofessional Partnerships

"In this inspiring book, Eisler and Potter show us why health care systems are changing and why nurses should have a leading role in this change. This book is a real gift for all the nurses in the world."

–Jos de Blok, RN
Consultant, Founder, and CEO
Buurtzorg, Almelo, Netherlands

"Today, we are facing a crucial turning point in our health care system. Eisler and Potter give us the language and inspire the courage to actively deconstruct the old domination paradigm and form the new partnership paradigm. This book is an essential road map to creating a more healing and caring health care world."

–Mary Koloroutis, MSN, RN
Vice President and Senior Consultant
Creative Health Care Management

"The solution to transforming our struggling health care system is nothing less than a cultural and paradigm shift. Presently, physicians occupy the dominator position with other health care professionals supporting them. What is needed is a model of systemic interprofessional partnership between doctors and nurses. With scholarly expertise and literary grace, Riane Eisler and Teddie Potter demonstrate exactly how this shift can happen. I loved this illuminating, inspiring book."

–Bill Manahan, MD
Past President, American Holistic Medical Association
Assistant Professor Emeritus, Department of Family Medicine
University of Minnesota Academic Health Center
Author of Eat for Health: Fast and Simple Ways of Eliminating Diseases Without Medical Advice

"*Transforming Interprofessional Partnerships* by Eisler and Potter illuminates the patterns of domination that have constrained the nursing profession. They insightfully offer that only by understanding the patterns of the past is there hope for shaping a different future. Their partnership framework represents a bold and dramatic shift from hierarchies of domination to high-functioning, interprofessional teams that will be poised and prepared to be full partners with patients, families, communities, and each other. Readers will appreciate the concrete and practical steps that are offered on how to embody the partnership principles in education, research, and practice."

–*Mary Jo Kreitzer, PhD, RN, FAAN*
Director, Center for Spirituality & Healing
Professor, School of Nursing
University of Minnesota

"Eisler and Potter have done a brilliant job of mapping the wisdom of the past and charting a course for the future through the exploration of a partnership paradigm. They provide insights, tools, and strategies about the power and promise of nursing medicine and of the tensions between domination and partnership. Reading this book is likely to shift the consciousness of health care providers and the public and spark a revolution toward a caring economy."

–*Daniel J Pesut, PhD, RN, PMHCNS-BC, FAAN, ACC*
Professor of Nursing Population Health and Systems Cooperative Unit
Director, Katharine Densford International Center for Nursing Leadership
Katherine R. and C. Walton Lillehei Chair in Nursing Leadership
University of Minnesota School of Nursing

"Attempts at interprofessional education (IPE) are waffling, missing a grounded 'what and why' of the aim. Eisler and Potter's book launches a dialogue required of all who are involved with IPE. Readers will resonate with this intelligent and theoretically intact book, with its cultural, professional, historic, and multinational narratives. In elucidating medicine and nursing paradigms, collaboration sans domination could advance an era of action-oriented decision science, enhancing holistic clinical outcomes. This is the purpose of IPE."

–*Michael R. Bleich, PhD, RN, FAAN*
Maxine Clark and Bob Fox Dean and Professor
Goldfarb School of Nursing, Barnes-Jewish College

"This book is extremely timely in its contribution to the theoretical rigor of interprofessional practice and education. It is easily accessible, using narratives and reflections on history, prehistory, and cultural transformation to capture and hold the reader's attention. Illustrations of the dominance versus partnership dichotomy offer novel insights into the benefits of developing a partnership-based culture within health care and inter/intraprofessional education, with practical suggestions on how this may be achieved."

–*Sarah Hean, Associate Professor*
Bournemouth University, UK

Transforming Interprofessional Partnerships

A New Framework for Nursing and Partnership-Based Health Care

Riane Eisler, JD, PhD(h) and Teddie M. Potter, PhD, RN

 Sigma Theta Tau International
Honor Society of Nursing®

Sigma Theta Tau International
Honor Society of Nursing®

The Honor Society of Nursing, Sigma Theta Tau International (STTI) is a nonprofit organization whose mission is to support the learning, knowledge, and professional development of nurses committed to making a difference in health worldwide. Founded in 1922, STTI has 130,000 members in 86 countries. Members include practicing nurses, instructors, researchers, policymakers, entrepreneurs and others. STTI's 486 chapters are located throughout Australia, Botswana, Brazil, Canada, Colombia, England, Ghana, Hong Kong, Japan, Kenya, Malawi, Mexico, Netherlands, Pakistan, Singapore, South Africa, South Korea, Swaziland, Sweden, Taiwan, Tanzania, the United States, and Wales. More information about STTI can be found online at www.nursingsociety.org.

Sigma Theta Tau International
550 West North Street
Indianapolis, IN, USA 46202

To order additional books, buy in bulk, or order for corporate use, contact Nursing Knowledge International at 888.NKI.4YOU (888.654.4968/US and Canada) or +1.317.634.8171 (outside US and Canada).

To request a review copy for course adoption, email solutions@nursingknowledge.org or call 888.NKI.4YOU (888.654.4968/US and Canada) or +1.317.917.4983 (outside US and Canada).

To request author information, or for speaker or other media requests, contact Marketing, the Honor Society of Nursing, Sigma Theta Tau International at 888.634.7575 (US and Canada) or +1.317.634.8171 (outside US and Canada).

ISBN:	9781938835261
EPUB ISBN:	9781938835278
PDF ISBN:	9781938835285
MOBI ISBN:	9781938835292

Library of Congress Cataloging-in-Publication Data

Eisler, Riane Tennenhaus, author.
 Transforming interprofessional partnerships : a new framework for nursing and partnership-based health care / Riane Eisler, Teddie M. Potter.
    p. ; cm.
Includes bibliographical references.
ISBN 978-1-938835-26-1 (book : alk. paper) -- ISBN 978-1-938835-27-8 (ePUB) -- ISBN 978-1-938835-28-5 (PDF) -- ISBN 978-1-938835-29-2 (MOBI)
I. Potter, Teddie M., 1956- author. II. Sigma Theta Tau International, publisher. III. Title.
[DNLM: 1. Advanced Practice Nursing--methods. 2. Interprofessional Relations. 3. Education, Nursing--methods. 4. Nursing Research--methods. 5. Public-Private Sector Partnerships. 6. Transcultural Nursing. WY 88]
RT86.54
362.17'3--dc23
                        2013042813

First Printing, 2014

Publisher: Renee Wilmeth	Principal Book Editor: Carla Hall
Acquisitions Editor: Emily Hatch	Development and Project Editor: Kevin Kent
Editorial Coordinator: Paula Jeffers	Copy Editor: Tonya Maddox Cupp
Cover Designer: Kim Scott @ Bumpy Design	Proofreader: Andrew Kimmel
Interior Design/Page Layout: Katy Bodenmiller	Indexer: Jane Palmer

Dedication

"Nurses should be full partners, with physicians and other health care professionals, in redesigning health care in the United States."

—Institute of Medicine (IOM),
The Future of Nursing: Leading Change,
Advancing Health, 2010

To my children and grandchildren, and to David, my wonderful partner.

—Riane

To Mom and Dad, who laid a strong and steady foundation for my life by raising me in a hierarchy of actualization, and to my dear Stephen, who furthers my knowledge and appreciation of partnership every day.

—Teddie

To all current and future nurses dedicated to making partnership-based health care a reality.

—Riane and Teddie

Acknowledgments

First and foremost, I want to thank Teddie for proposing that we write this book together, and for being such a wonderful partner in doing so.

I also want to thank the nurses I met in person when I keynoted the University of Minnesota nursing conference, the Summit of Sages, and the nurses I met online through our Center for Partnership Studies webinars. They too have enriched my understanding of nursing and health care.

Working with Teddie on this book has given me the opportunity to apply my research and thinking to areas that are extremely important, not only for the healing professions, but for us all. Indeed, working on this book has been an opportunity to learn and to expand my thinking, and for this I am most grateful.

–Riane

I have come to believe if we are open to ideas and willing to venture where others have not gone before, we won't write a book; the book will write us. This book is no exception, taking on a life of its own as I explored past and present thinking about partnership and interprofessional practice. New ideas and nursing theories evolved as gaps in the current interprofessional curriculum became evident.

The journey of writing this book was both meaningful and enjoyable thanks to my traveling partners. I would like to thank my students in the Doctor of Nursing Practice in Health Innovation and Leadership specialty at the University of Minnesota. You have been both willing subjects and a source of inspiration as I tried out new models and ways of thinking. Through your partnership-based quality improvement projects you have demonstrated that partnership-based health care is more than a dream; it is an effective and sustainable paradigm capable of transforming health care today.

I want to thank our community partners who have generously shared their time and materials, including the Institute for Patient- and Family-Centered Care, Marie Manthey and Creative Health Care Management, and *Buurtzorg Nederland*.

Last but not least, I want to acknowledge Riane's profound gift of agreeing to be my mentor and role model. She has dedicated her entire life to creating a healthier society, and health care professionals will surely benefit from her theories.

–Teddie

We both want to express our thanks for the support of our editorial team at Sigma Theta Tau International, especially Emily Hatch, Kevin Kent, Carla Hall, and all the others who have worked on this book, whose enthusiasm and helpfulness added yet another positive dimension to our joint work.

–Riane and Teddie

About the Authors

Riane Eisler, JD, PhD(h)

Riane Eisler is internationally known for her contributions as a systems scientist, attorney working for the human rights of women and children, and author of *The Chalice and the Blade: Our History, Our Future* (1987), now in 25 foreign editions, and *The Real Wealth of Nations: Creating a Caring Economics* (2007), hailed by Archbishop Desmond Tutu as "a template for the better world we have been so urgently seeking."

Eisler is founder and president of the Center for Partnership Studies, dedicated to research, education, and public policy work through programs such as the Spiritual Alliance to Stop Intimate Violence (SAIV), which Eisler co-founded with Nobel Peace laureate Betty Williams, and the Caring Economy Campaign, which shows the financial value of policies and practices that invest in people and nature.

She consults for business and governments on practical applications of the partnership model introduced in her work and keynotes conferences and speaks at universities and corporations internationally, with venues including the United Nations General Assembly, the U.S. Department of State, congressional briefings, and events hosted by heads of State such as Rita Suessmuth, former president of the German parliament, and Vaclav Havel, former president of the Czech Republic.

She is a member of the Club of Rome, a councilor of the World Future Council and the International Museum of Women, a fellow of the Academy of Art and Science and the World Business Academy, a commissioner of the World Commission on Global Consciousness and Spirituality, and a member of other international and national councils. She has taught at UCLA and now teaches in the Leadership graduate program at the California Institute of Integral Studies. In addition to the two books mentioned earlier, she is author of the award-winning books *Tomorrow's Children: A Blueprint for Partnership Education in the 21st Century* and *The Power of Partnership: Seven Relationships That Will Change*

Your Life, as well as *Sacred Pleasure: Sex, Myth, and the Politics of the Body,* a daring reexamination of sexuality and spirituality, and *Women, Men, and the Global Quality of Life,* documenting the key role of women's status in a nation's general quality of life. She has written over 400 articles in publications ranging from *Behavioral Science, Challenge, Political Psychology, Brain and Mind, Christian Science Monitor,* to *The UNESCO Courier to the Human Rights Quarterly,* the *International Journal of Women's Studies, Futures,* and the *World Encyclopedia of Peace.*

She has received many honors, including honorary PhD degrees and the Nuclear Age Peace Foundation's 2009 Distinguished Peace Leadership Award, and is included in the award-winning book *Great Peacemakers* as one of 20 leaders for world peace, along with Mahatma Gandhi, Mother Teresa, and Dr. Martin Luther King, Jr.

Teddie M. Potter, PhD, RN

Teddie Potter has a long history of being at the heart of paradigm shifts, including being one of the first home care nurses in her state, starting a specialized home care program for people living with HIV/AIDS, and helping start one of the first palliative care programs in the nation. She has also shown a long-term commitment to diversity and inclusivity, studying factors that help diverse students succeed in nursing school and teaching healing traditions of our diverse community.

Her current positions in the School of Nursing at the University of Minnesota are a natural extension of her interests and passions. She is clinical associate professor and coordinator of the Doctor of Nursing Practice in Health Innovation and Leadership program and director of Inclusivity and Diversity.

Her global travels and deep concern for the health of the environment have led her to believe that our current path, based on domination principles and values, is not compatible with health and life on this planet. Therefore, she is deeply committed to further development of theories and curricula that support effective and sustainable partnership-based health care.

Table of Contents

Foreword

Throughout the course of my career, certain books have appeared at points in time that profoundly challenged my thinking and, at the same time, were so familiar to inner truths that I had not yet put into words. The first was Carol Gilligan's *In a Different Voice* (1982), which examined the voices and viewpoints of women and offered a new way of thinking about relationships and responsibility and how women make choices and pursue their goals. The second book appeared in 1992—Meg Wheatley's *Leadership and the New Science: Discovering Order in a Chaotic World*. This book transformed our thinking about leading organizations, asserting that the previous approach of trying to exert more control over chaos was failing. There is a "simpler way," and it is based on relationships and transparency.

The third book is Riane Eisler and Teddie Potter's *Transforming Interprofessional Partnerships: A New Framework for Nursing and Partnership-Based Health Care*. As with the other two books, it shatters historical patterns of thought, in this case the inevitability of the domination model of relationships. It describes what has come to be an accepted way of life, which has marginalized or silenced knowing voices, and points to a better way that invites inclusion and inspires hope. All three of these books address the power of relationships and offer a different way of thinking about contemporary issues at a level that is *truly* a paradigm shift. They all challenge our assumptions and beliefs.

However, Eisler and Potter also provide a map for our journey and a framework. With *Transforming Interprofessional Partnerships*, the authors draw from a wide range of fields of study, such as archeology, mythology, history, sociology, psychology, and economics, and offer examples over thousands of years to illustrate their key points. They offer a shared language and concepts that apply broadly. Concepts such as relational dynamics, cultural transformation, hierarchies of actualization, and caring economics are explored in the context of nursing today. Their discussion of the "medicine of nursing" is brilliant, and the model that is the "BASE of Nursing" can guide nursing practice in any setting and nursing education in any program.

To help us on the journey of becoming more aware and skilled at establishing partnership relationships, this book provides exemplars, innovative teaching strategies, and practical suggestions. Within each chapter, there is a rich compilation of relevant studies and resources for further reading. From a personal standpoint, the book provokes total reflection on one's own beliefs and practices. What examples of domination or partnership have I witnessed or experienced? Are there any that I have unwittingly contributed to? What do my words convey? What can I do better? A goal of theirs is to help nurses strengthen their sense of self-identity but also to be stronger partners in interprofessional practice, education, and research endeavors. An implicit thread throughout the book is working with others and better understanding oneself.

For all of the above reasons, I will return to this book often. In Eisler and Potter's own words, this "book breaks new ground. At the same time, it reclaims old wisdoms and insights" (p. xx). In addition to the helpful frameworks, concepts, and strategies, it also has served as an inspiring and heartening reminder of nursing's sources of power, our shared strengths, and the wisdom and tenacity of some of our early leaders.

–Joanne Disch, PhD, RN, FAAN
Clinical Professor, University of Minnesota School of Nursing

References

Gilligan, C. (1982). *In a different voice: Psychological theory and women's development.* Cambridge, MA: Harvard University Press.

Wheatley, M.J. (1992). *Leadership and the new science: Discovering order in a chaotic world.* San Francisco, CA: Berrett-Koehler.

Introduction

"The most remarkable feature of this historical moment on Earth is not that we are on the way to destroying the world—we've actually been on the way for quite a while. It is that we are beginning to wake up, as from a millennia-long sleep, to a whole new relationship to our world, to ourselves and to each other."

—Joanna Macy, 2012

Many of us are becoming aware that old ways of thinking cannot help us effectively meet our unprecedented personal, social, and economic challenges. Ours is a historic time when people worldwide are trying to reawaken the full potential of new relationships, not only with one another, but also with ourselves. This is why we hear so much today about a shift to a new paradigm, to a new way of seeing ourselves and our world.

This shift in paradigms is especially important for the nursing profession, which has for far too long labored under a paradigm in which nursing's unique contribution to healing has been marginalized. This marginalization has narrowed our vision and limited our practice, with very negative implications not only for our health care systems, but also for all our lives.

The goal of this book is to provide nurses and other health care professionals tools to reexamine what we were often taught is "just the way things are" and to build a more effective, caring, and sustainable health care system.

In cowriting this book, we have drawn from each of our life experiences, both personally and professionally. We have also drawn from a large body of research, both our own and that of many others: research that both deconstructs the old paradigm and provides building blocks for a new paradigm that in bits and pieces is trying to come together, albeit against resistance and periodic regressions.

In significant respects this book breaks new ground. At the same time, it reclaims old wisdoms and insights. It brings together knowledge from many disciplines and places nursing and health care in their larger historical and social context. Above all, it offers a roadmap to a better future, not only for nursing and health care, but also for all who seek a healthier path.

An Introduction to Paradigms and New Thinking

In 1962, physicist and philosopher Thomas Kuhn wrote *The Structure of Scientific Revolutions*, which describes the revolutionary nature of scientific knowledge. Instead of being a linear process, the evolution of knowledge tends to come in bursts of clarity, which occur in response to anomalies. *Anomalies* are phenomena that cannot be explained by the current set of assumptions and provide irreconcilable evidence that the existing paradigm no longer works.

Kuhn's 1962 work also recognizes that knowledge acquisition is a communal process, with the scientific community often coming together to embrace new ways of thinking. Kuhn coined the term *paradigm shift* to describe this phenomenon. In science, classic examples of paradigm shifts include the Copernican revolution, Einstein's theory of relativity, and the rise of quantum physics.

Kuhn did not relate these scientific paradigm shifts to changes in society. However, if you broaden your lens of analysis, you can see that these shifts in thinking did not happen in a vacuum. They were each part of larger social changes—changes that, as you see in this book, were attempts to shift from a *domination system* to a *partnership system*. For example, the Copernican scientific revolution, which was considered a heresy by those in power, occurred at a time when rigid theocratic rule was beginning to be challenged. Einstein's theory of relativity came at a time when many other absolutes—dogmas about what is or is not natural or divinely ordained—were being challenged, including the "natural" or "divinely ordained superiority" of one kind of group over another. Quantum physics was a scientific manifestation of a growing recognition of the interconnection of all life—in other words, of movement toward a more partnership-oriented paradigm.

In sum, paradigm shifts in science—and as you read in this book, in health care—do not happen in isolation. They are part of a larger shift in stories about what *is,* or *is not,* normal or abnormal, possible or impossible.

Our Stories

This takes us to another set of stories we want to briefly share with you before we begin to look at the paradigm shift in our health care systems. These are our own stories, which are relevant not only so you know where we are coming from, but also because they illustrate the process of paradigm change—and its real-life results.

Teddie's Story

In 1979, with a great deal of enthusiasm and a deep commitment to the work of health care, I launched my nursing career. For 3 years, first on the East Coast and then in the Midwest, I worked in acute care. Even though my second job was on a unit that used the primary care nursing model, I still had numerous humiliating physician-nurse experiences. Gradually I became conscious that the old top-down model of care not only harms nurses, but also directly impacts the quality and safety of patients.

Then came a number of other important changes in my consciousness. In 1983, I transferred to home care, an emerging health care delivery model that would end up being my practice setting for the next 3 decades. Home care offers nurses more autonomy and is a natural setting for patient- and family-centered care. The non-local nature of home care also necessitates respectful nurse-physician relationships. I became aware of the advantages of these kinds of relationships for all concerned.

My experiences in hospice home care gave me a wonderful opportunity to be part of an effective interprofessional team. I did not know it at the time, but what I experienced in the first 5 years of my career is the difference between domination-based and partnership-based models of health care.

I have always been interested in paradigm shifts and the changes in consciousness they entail. So in 1988, I picked up a copy of Riane Eisler's (1987)

The Chalice and the Blade: Our History, Our Future. Little did I know when I started to read this book that it would become a major influence in my practice and my life. *The Chalice and the Blade* not only helped me name and understand the two different paradigms I had experienced, but also helped me understand that throughout history people have had a choice of assumptions and principles on which to base their relationships. That meant I no longer was a victim of my cultural story. I too could choose which paradigm I wanted to use to guide my personal and professional life.

Eventually I felt called to return to school and earn my master's in nursing so I could teach. Like all creative teachers, I tried my ideas out in curriculum design and clinical mentorship with my students. The results were beyond my wildest dreams. A partnership approach to teaching stimulated the growth and development of students, empowering them to be lifelong learners and full partners with patients and other health care professionals.

But I wanted to know more about the partnership paradigm and how I could bring about a shift in health care education and practice. Then I made the decision to attend the California Institute of Integral Studies (CIIS) for my PhD education because at some level I recognized that my inquiry would likely require both a transdisciplinary and integral approach. Imagine my surprise and delight at orientation when I learned one of the new adjunct professors at CIIS was Riane Eisler!

At CIIS, I had the amazing opportunity to take courses directly from Riane, and, as I did, my unique research question came into focus. I wanted to know which factors limit the practice of nurses and how nurses can be empowered to reach their fullest potential. I came to believe Eisler's research provides the theory and principles for a necessary shift in health care; yet her work had not been used in either nursing or health care. I had discovered the gap that aligned with my personal goals and vision.

In my dissertation, *Reconstructing a New Story of Nursing: Critical Analysis of Nursing Textbooks* using Riane Eisler's *Partnership Paradigm* (Potter, 2010), I connected Eisler's cultural transformation theory to nursing and health care. I was further delighted when Riane agreed to serve on my dissertation committee.

As nursing faculty, I saw two repetitive themes: There is an education-practice gap related to partnership-based health care, and there is a severe shortage of resources to help health care providers move the health care system toward partnership. One morning I woke up, quickly grabbed the nearest paper and pen, and jotted down the framework for this book.

If I had still adhered to the rigid hierarchies of the domination paradigm, I never would have had the courage to bring my book idea to Riane. But my experiences as her graduate student were of mutual respect and open communication—and by then I had become a devoted disciple of partnership and hierarchies of actualization. Therefore, I did not hesitate to contact Riane with the idea for this book. And the rest, as they say, is history.

Riane's Story

My story too is one of major changes in consciousness—which, in my life, started very early with a number of traumatic events. I was born in Vienna at a time that in terms of the conceptual framework of the *partnership/domination continuum* was a major regression to domination: the rise to power of the Nazis, first in Germany and then in my native Austria. On November 10, 1938—later known as Crystal Night because so much glass was shattered in Jewish stores, homes, and synagogues—a gang of Nazis came for my father, shoved him down the stairs, and dragged him off.

I watched in horror as consciousness of the reality of cruelty and violence was etched into my developing brain. But almost at the same time, I became conscious of something equally powerful: the reality of love and of courage, of what I today call *spiritual courage*—the courage to stand up against injustice out of love. When my mother recognized one of the Gestapo men as a former errand boy for the family business, she furiously upbraided him for his brutal treatment of a man who had been kind to him and demanded my father's release.

My mother could have been killed; the Nazis killed many people that night. But miraculously she instead obtained my father's release, and after some money changed hands, my parents and I were able to flee to Paris, and later to Cuba.

My experiences in Cuba too were traumatic. Uprooted from all that was familiar, we were plunged into brutal poverty, as my parents had to leave everything they owned behind when we fled. It was also growing up in the industrial slums of Havana that I later learned that most of our relatives—grandparents, aunts, uncles, and cousins—had been killed in Nazi concentration camps during the Holocaust, which would have happened to us had we not escaped by a hair's breadth.

These experiences led me to burning questions: Why is there so much cruelty, destructiveness, and injustice in the world? Is this our inevitable lot? Or can we create a more peaceful, just, and caring world?

Over the years, I looked for answers to these questions in books and universities, but never found satisfactory ones. Then I took a job as a social scientist at the Systems Development Corporation, an offshoot of the Rand Corporation, where I learned a basic principle of systems thinking: Looking at how different parts of a system interact makes it possible to see more than the system's parts.

That was in the 1950s, and many things happened before I returned to the questions of my childhood. I married, had two lovely daughters, went back to school to obtain a law degree in addition to my degree in sociology, got a divorce, became involved in the civil rights and then the women's movements, and used my legal training to change unjust and discriminatory laws.

But after a while I saw that while changing laws is essential, it is not enough, and that what is needed is a fundamental paradigm shift. By then it was the 1970s, and it was becoming evident that using violence to settle international disputes in our age of nuclear and biological weapons was unsustainable. Also clear was that advanced technologies in service of the once-hallowed conquest of nature were causing environmental damage of unprecedented, potentially lethal, dimensions.

So I went back to my training in social and systems science and embarked on the multidisciplinary study of our past, present, and the possibilities for our future that eventually led to another major change in my consciousness. I realized that I could not answer my questions by looking at societies through the lenses of conventional social categories such as religious versus secular, rightist versus leftist, Eastern versus Western, capitalist versus socialist, and so on; societies in all these categories have been repressive and violent. I then made the discovery through my research that transcending these differences are two basic social configurations: the partnership system and the domination system.

This discovery changed not only my consciousness but also that of many others through my books (including *The Chalice and the Blade*, which is now in 25 foreign editions), articles, classes, and speeches, as well as through the books, articles, classes, and speeches of others using the findings from my research in addition to their own.

One of these people is my coauthor and former student, Teddie Potter, who has applied this work in both her teaching and writing about nursing, and with whom it has been a great pleasure to write this book on how cultural transformation theory can help move health care to a more effective, sustainable model by empowering nurses and other health care professionals to actively bring forth partnership-based health care.

Invitation to Health Care Professionals

Throughout this book you will see how the story and experience of the nursing profession illustrate the differences between the domination and partnership paradigms. You will see that many of the assumptions guiding current health care systems are obstacles to forward movement and need to be replaced. You will also see how the tension between the partnership and domination configuration has historically impacted every health care profession.

We therefore invite you to read this book with your own professional narrative in mind. We invite you to use this book's framework to help your own profession see how it has been limited and disempowered by the traditional domination-based model of health care.

As you read, ask yourself these questions:

- What is my profession's unique medicine?

- How have threads of domination and partnership played out in the history of my profession?

- How can my profession teach students to be full partners in interprofessional practice?

- How can I be a full partner with colleagues from within my profession? How can I be an effective intraprofessional colleague?

- What can my profession do to foster partnership with other health care professionals, with patients and families, and with communities?

- How can my profession further the paradigm shift toward partnership and a caring economics model?

Ultimately a shift from domination to partnership will require the participation of each and every one of us. This book offers all of us a map for our journey.

The Contents of This Book

This text provides the framework to shift health care relationships from hierarchies of domination and isolated professions to high-functioning interprofessional teams ready to be full partners with patients, families, communities, and one another.

Part I introduces a common language.

Chapter 1 challenges the domination-based assumption that only one profession makes a contribution to medicine or to the process of healing. Through the narrative lens of nursing, the chapter offers a new practice and research model—the BASE of Nursing (Potter, 2013) to support an expanded understanding of medicine.

Chapter 2 gives a brief overview of the emerging field of interprofessional education and collaborative practice (IPECP). This overview provides the rationale for partnership-based education and practice.

Part II deconstructs the old cultural narrative, making room for a new cultural story.

Chapter 3 is an in-depth description of Eisler's (1987, 2002) cultural transformation theory (CTT).

In **Chapter 4,** Potter uses CTT to identify patterns of domination in the recorded history of nursing.

Then, in **Chapter 5,** Potter uses the lived experience of a number of important historic nurses to give nurses an alternative partnership-based narrative. This new narrative can help nurses reclaim an empowered identity and prepare them to be full partners in interprofessional practice.

Part III offers readers a template to shift every relationship in health care toward partnership.

Chapter 6 begins with professional education. Because this is where socialization to our professional roles is initiated, it is critical to ensure that curricula include partnership values and principles.

Chapter 7 discusses these important domains. When nurses and other novice health care professionals start their practice, one of their most important relationships will be with themselves. Professional identity and self-care are critical aspects of effective interprofessional practice.

Chapter 8 initiates a discussion of how to partner with those we serve. This chapter discusses patient- and family-centered care and how to support this partnership-based model.

In **Chapter 9,** we challenge intraprofessional incivility or harmful and disempowering relationships within a profession. If we do not adequately identify the abuse of rank and peer-to-peer lateral violence, we are unlikely to function appropriately in interprofessional teams.

Chapter 10 offers a vision for partnership-based interprofessional practice. It moves us beyond simply collaborating to an empowering model that supports full partnership and engagement of all health care professionals.

Chapter 11 applies partnership principles to care in the community, showing how partnership-based interprofessional teams can make a difference in all environments, from the hospital bedside to clinics, health care homes, and other emerging models of community-centered care.

The final chapter of this section, **Chapter 12,** questions assumptions about nature and healing that we inherited from more rigid domination times. It also offers partnership alternatives to the old conquest-of-nature perspective.

Part IV acknowledges that a national and global shift toward partnership-based health care requires a shift in our economic models.

Chapter 13, therefore, introduces Riane Eisler's (2007) caring economics model—a new economic model that supports the critical work of caring for others.

In **Chapter 14,** we conclude this book with an invitation to our readers to join together to shift health care toward partnership. We offer specific steps that we can all take to identify and challenge threads of domination in our personal lives, our professional work, and in how we teach and model a partnership perspective in education, practice, and research. We show that changes are possible, that they are already being made, and that we can each play a part to ensure we all reach our full potential as healers, individuals, and communities.

References

Eisler, R. (1987). *The chalice and the blade: Our history, our future.* San Francisco, CA: HarperCollins.

Eisler, R. (2002). *The power of partnership: Seven relationships that will change your life.* Novato, CA: New World Publishing.

Eisler, R. (2007). *The real wealth of nations: Creating a caring economics.* San Francisco, CA: Berret-Koehler.

Institute of Medicine (IOM). (2010). *The future of nursing: Leading change, advancing health.* Washington, DC: National Academies.

Kuhn, T. S. (1970). *The structure of scientific revolutions.* Chicago, IL: University of Chicago Press.

Macy, J. (2012). The great turning. Retrieved from http://www.joannamacy.net/

Potter, T. M. (2010). Reconstructing a new story of nursing: Critical analysis of nursing textbooks using Riane Eisler's partnership paradigm. *Dissertation Abstracts International, 72*(05), 3447086.

Potter, T. M. (2013). *The BASE of nursing.* Unpublished manuscript, School of Nursing, University of Minnesota, United States of America.

Part I
Creating a Shared Identity

"The single biggest problem in communication is the illusion that it has taken place."

–George Bernard Shaw

If nurses are to be full partners with patients, other health professionals, and even one another, we must be able to communicate a shared professional identity and a common understanding of our unique contribution to interprofessional practice.

Chapter 1 expands the definition of medicine, returning to its original Latin meaning as "the art of healing or making whole." This perspective of medicine allows nurses to come to interprofessional practice as equals, recognizing that we all bring medicine to the care of patients, families, and communities.

Effective communication for interprofessional practice requires every health care professional to have a strong professional identity. All professionals need to fully understand and appreciate their roles and responsibilities on the health care team and the nature of their unique medicine or contribution in helping patients, families, and communities reach wholeness. To this end, Chapter 1 introduces the *BASE of Nursing* (Potter, 2013), a new nursing paradigm that illuminates nursing's unique medicine.

Chapter 2 then introduces readers to the history, theory, language, and principles of interprofessional education and collaborative practice (IPECP). This chapter allows both newcomers and experts to the field of interprofessional education and practice to share a language and common knowledge of where the field has been and where it may be going.

Through these two chapters, Part I lays a foundation and establishes the context for preparing health care providers to work together to cocreate partnership-based health care.

Chapter 1
The Medicine of Nursing

"To build a partnership culture we need to reexamine beliefs, myths, and stories—strengthening those that promote partnership and discarding those that do not."

–Riane Eisler (2002, p. 219)

It is time for an expanded understanding of medicine. A powerful and pervasive myth in biomedical health care systems is that the domain of medicine belongs solely to physicians. A more inclusive definition of medicine creates a shared language for partnership-based interprofessional education (IPE) and interprofessional practice (IPP). It also creates a shared language for the global health care community. Partnerships frequently come together around a shared goal or common cause. Physicians, nurses, and other health providers share many aspects of knowledge and practice. The common goal of all health care professions is the *appropriate and effective use of medicine to promote, sustain, and recover health.*

The word *medicine* may appear to make this statement only applicable to physicians. However, sole ownership of the concept of medicine poses one of the greatest challenges to effective interprofessional partnerships. A more inclusive understanding is that each health care profession has proprietorship over its own medicine. Indeed, effective interprofessional practice is possible only when each profession's unique medicine is respected and empowered to reach its full potential.

What Is Medicine?

The word *medicine* is derived from the Latin word *medicina*, which can be translated as "the art of healing," with *healing* defined as "to make whole" (Heal, n.d.). In ancient times, medicine or the art of healing was practiced by diverse providers including herbalists, animists, shamans, and bonesetters. Male and female healers since the dawn of time have practiced medicine every time they provided care that alleviated suffering.

If you consider the scope of human history, the physician's claim to the domain of medicine is a rather new phenomenon. In Western Europe during the 13th century, the secular science of medicine began to dominate after it was taught in universities. Females who were forbidden enrollment in all-male universities were effectively denied formal education in medicine (Ehrenreich & English, 1973). The relationship among power, gender, and nursing history will be discussed further in Chapter 4.

Nonetheless, the United States was slow to adopt a medicine monopoly. It wasn't until 1848, when the American Medical Association (AMA) was established and gained sufficient power, that science-based medicine was claimed to be the "true" medicine (Ehrenreich & English, 1973). By the early 20th century, other forms of medicine such as homeopathic medicine, herbal medicine, osteopathic medicine, and chiropractic medicine began to be marginalized and dismissed as quackery (Getzendanner, 1988; Loudon, 2006; Reeves & Burke, 2009).

Biomedicine, or science-based medicine, is also a relatively new system of medicine. Many ancient systems of medicine still exist and are used by billions of people around the globe. Examples include traditional Chinese medicine, Ayurvedic medicine of India, and indigenous systems of medicine around the globe. Globalization and expansion of knowledge via the Internet are pushing more people to redefine the domain of medicine and argue for a blending or integration of the best healing methods.

Is There a Medicine of Nursing?

Starting with the definition that medicine is the "art of healing," we see that any health care profession that aims to heal or "make whole" has a right to claim it has a unique practice of medicine. Nursing is often associated with providing care under doctor's orders, but independent nursing interventions definitely contribute to patient healing or wholeness as well. Therefore, there is a unique medicine of nursing.

For much of the nursing profession's modern history, people have been told that a nurse's primary role is to administer the medicine of physicians. Consequently, nursing care is frequently pushed into the shadows in a hierarchy that ranks one profession's medicine over another. And in many ways, nursing education has been complicit in supporting this myth by its increased emphasis on the biomedical model.

Expanding our awareness to recognize the medicine of nursing requires a disciplined mind. An expanded understanding of medicine helps everyone see that physicians and nurses contribute both shared and unique knowledge to health care. Shared areas of medicine include knowledge based on the scientific method. Nurses and physicians also share similar ethical values, including non-maleficence and beneficence. In addition, many nurses and physicians also believe that our minds, bodies, and spirits impact both health and illness. And most physicians, nurses, and other health care providers are motivated by care and concern for people. Just as physicians do not own the domain of medicine, nurses do not own the domain of caring.

NURSE AND PHYSICIAN AREAS OF SHARED MEDICINE

Both nurses and physicians:

- *Care about the patient*

- *Are concerned about the physical condition of the patient*

- *Conduct initial assessments that include:*

  - *Subjective data: Chief concern, history of present illness, past medical history, family history, social history, including risk factors and current lifestyle*

  - *Objective data: Head-to-toe assessment or review of systems*

- *Analyze the data: Determine the problem, list potential diagnoses (medical or nursing) causing the acute problem or describe the status of a chronic problem, and support the conclusion with clinical reasoning or evidence*

- *Perform evidence-based interventions*

- *Evaluate responses to interventions and treatments*

- *Work collaboratively with other health professionals*

- *Document care and treatments*

- *Participate in ongoing professional development to maintain licensure or certification*

- *Participate in professional organizations, and conduct and disseminate research to advance knowledge in the profession*

- *Have an orientation toward service, a specialized body of knowledge, practical and theoretical education, autonomy, knowledge based on scientific research, representation by a professional organization, an extended period of education, ongoing professional development, and standards of practice to guide their profession*

Additionally, registered nurses and physicians develop a treatment plan, do patient education, and plan for follow-up. Both advanced practice registered nurses and physicians can order diagnostic testing and prescribe pharmaceuticals.

Yet nursing *does* have a unique system of medicine. This unique medicine is the process by which nurses create wholeness.

How do nurses heal or make whole? According to the American Nurses Association (ANA), "Nursing is the protection, promotion, and optimization of health and abilities, prevention of illness and injury, alleviation of suffering through the diagnosis and treatment of human response, and advocacy in the care of individuals, families, communities, and populations" (ANA, 2013). Although this statement includes what nurses do, it does not fully capture what it means to *be* a nurse.

The International Council of Nurses (ICN) has a somewhat more comprehensive definition of nursing:

> *Nursing encompasses autonomous and collaborative care of individuals of all ages, families, groups and communities, sick or well and in all settings. Nursing includes the promotion of health, prevention of illness, and the care of ill, disabled and dying people. Advocacy, promotion of a safe environment, research, participation in shaping health policy and in patient and health systems management, and education are also key nursing roles. (ICN, 2010)*

Once again, this statement defines nursing by roles, and all the roles it enumerates overlap with the medicine of others, including physicians and social workers. Rather than using roles, a professional nursing paradigm can more clearly define the unique medicine of nursing.

A number of scholars have recognized that a well-defined nursing identity or paradigm is essential for effective interdisciplinary work. For instance, Castledine (2005) suggested that "nurses need to be more confident of their nursing work, its origins, and purpose" to ensure successful interprofessional collaboration (p. 3). However, as Benner, Sutphen, Leonard, and Day reported in 2010, many nurses lack clarity about their purpose, given the role ambiguity in today's health care environment. This lack of clarity is symptomatic of the problem of identity of nurses.

For example, Cowin (2001) found little agreement in the literature about the elements of nursing identity—even though a sense of identity strongly correlates with job satisfaction, stress, burnout, and attrition levels. When nursing identity has been discussed, the traditional paradigm tied it to four domains: person, environment, health, and nursing. This model however, fails to encompass some specialties such as public health nursing, nursing administration or leadership, and nursing informatics. The current nursing paradigm also strongly emphasizes evidence-based practice. But commitment to only one domain fails to describe the full breadth and depth of nursing knowledge and nursing care (Cull-Wilby & Pepin, 1987).

Some more recent nursing textbooks attempt to address these gaps by including presence, empowering the client, compassion, and competence as features of the unique nursing paradigm (Potter, 2010). These are important steps forward, but more is needed for a well-defined nursing identity appropriate for a health care paradigm in which the nursing profession is a full partner in interprofessional health care teams.

The BASE of Nursing Medicine

For nurses to discuss and advocate for nursing care, they must be able to articulate the full base of nursing's medicine. Potter's (2013) *BASE of Nursing* (Figure 1.1) offers a common understanding of nursing that will be used throughout this book. This common understanding is key to a comprehensive nursing paradigm and includes nurses from all levels of nursing education, all cultures, and all practice settings and specialties.

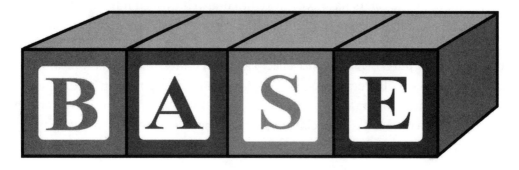

FIGURE 1.1 BASE OF NURSING.

All figures in this chapter are copyright S. Nesser. Used with permission.

The BASE of Nursing moves beyond evidence-based practice to a practice based on four domains: *Being* present, *Active* caring, *Stories/narratives*, and *Evidence* from science.

- B–Being present (Figure 1.2) represents the physical, emotional, and spiritual relationship that nurses have with patients, families, and/or communities.

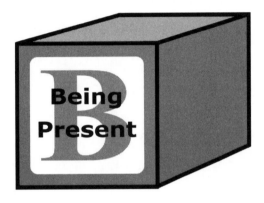

FIGURE 1.2 BEING PRESENT.

- A–Active caring (Figure 1.3) is the act of providing nursing care.

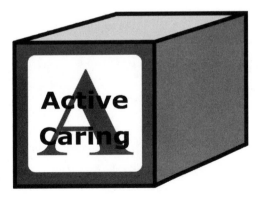

FIGURE 1.3 ACTIVE CARING.

- S–Stories (Figure 1.4) reflect narrative-based evidence, a form of knowledge obtained through the art of nursing. Stories are unique to the individual or the community, and therefore, narrative-based knowledge cannot be generalized.

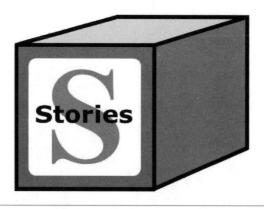

FIGURE 1.4 STORIES OR NARRATIVE-BASED EVIDENCE.

- E–Evidence from science (Figure 1.5), another way of saying evidence-based practice, is knowledge obtained through the science of nursing. This knowledge by definition is recognized by its generalizability.

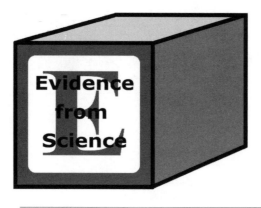

FIGURE 1.5 EVIDENCE FROM SCIENCE.

The BASE of Nursing (Potter, 2013) values all four domains and does not rank them hierarchically. It gives equal attention to relationship and knowledge, two important aspects of the medicine of nursing.

Ways of Relating

B and *A* (Figure 1.6) in the model reflect relationships—the way nurses interact with patients, families, and communities. Relationships can contain presence or action, or they may be a blend of both.

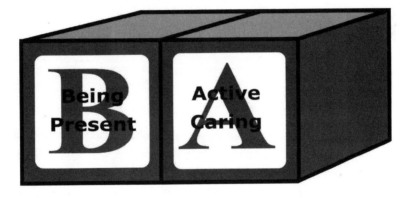

FIGURE 1.6 RELATIONSHIP.

Ways of Knowing

S and *E* (Figure 1.7) reflect sources of knowledge. Knowledge can be narrative-based or science-based, and both are equally valued aspects of the BASE of Nursing medicine.

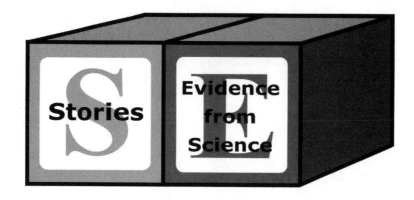

FIGURE 1.7 KNOWLEDGE.

Applying the BASE of Nursing

The four domains of the BASE of Nursing—being present, active caring, stories/narratives, and evidence from science—are interrelated and mutually supporting. Each domain has its own qualities or elements and is important in itself.

When Potter (2010) analyzed the autobiographies of several 19th and 20th century nurses, she found that these domains were common themes in their nursing as well. Note the italicized qualities in Figures 1.8–1.11; these qualities were mentioned in the autobiographies, demonstrating that these four domains have actually been integral to nursing for a long time.

Being Present

Therapeutic use of self or *being present* (Figure 1.8) is an essential principle of nursing medicine, and there is extensive nursing science supporting this domain.

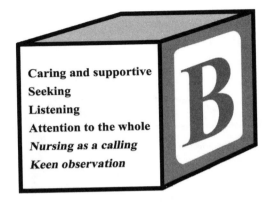

FIGURE 1.8 QUALITIES OF BEING PRESENT.

When McMahon and Christopher (2011) summarized studies on the use of presence in nursing, they found the following:

- Healing presence in nursing includes "knowing what will work and when to act" (p.73).

- Patient outcomes include clients that are "viewed as subjects not objects" and clients that "receive individualized care" (p. 73).

Fredriksson's (1999) synthesis of research on presence found, "The power of presence as 'being with' lies in making available a space where the patient can be in deep contact with his/her suffering, share it with a caring other, and find his/her own way forward" (p. 1171). Data also verify that healing or wholeness is facilitated by a nurse's deep physical, psychological, and spiritual presence with clients. More than simply being the way nursing medicine is administered, presence appears to be a significant aspect of nursing medicine. The act of being present is itself healing.

Active Caring

Active caring (Figure 1.9) in nursing takes many forms, from administration of medications to advocacy.

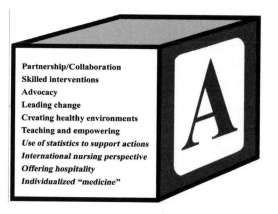

Partnership/Collaboration
Skilled interventions
Advocacy
Leading change
Creating healthy environments
Teaching and empowering
Use of statistics to support actions
International nursing perspective
Offering hospitality
Individualized "medicine"

FIGURE 1.9 QUALITIES OF ACTIVE CARING.

Hanks (2010) conducted a large survey of practicing medical surgical nurses and found participants most often defined advocacy as providing patient and family education, communicating with other health care team members, and questioning and ensuring adequate care for clients. Patient and family education empowers patients and increases their adherence to treatments. Communicating with other health professionals can yield improved patient quality outcomes, and questioning and ensuring adequate care can decrease errors and promote both safety and healing.

Active caring involves action and skilled ministration of dependent, independent, and collaborative interventions. It involves actions ranging from wound care to policy development. It affects all recipients, from individuals to systems.

As described by the Institute of Medicine (IOM), active caring requires nurses to "practice to the full extent of their education and training" (2010, p.3). Going even further, the IOM report *The Future of Nursing: Leading Change,*

Advancing Health states, "Nurses must act as full partners in redesign efforts, be accountable for their own contributions to delivering high-quality care, and work collaboratively with leaders from other health professions" (p. 3). Interprofessional partnerships are a major aspect of *active caring* in the nursing paradigm.

Stories/Narrative-Based Evidence

Nurses work with other health care providers, often making sure social determinants of health are considered. Nurses understand that individual wholeness or healing is compromised by unhealthy environments—be they social, economic, natural, or political. The ANA's *Holistic Nursing: Scope and Standards of Practice* (2007) states, "Holistic nurses (HNs) recognize the human health experience as a complicated, dynamic relationship of health, illness, and wellness, and they value healing as the desired outcome of the practice of nursing" (p. 65).

Compassionate concern for the whole person/environment relationship is therefore a fundamental part of nursing's medicine. And the key to understanding this "complicated and dynamic relationship of health, illness, and wellness" is stories, or narrative-based evidence (Figure 1.10).

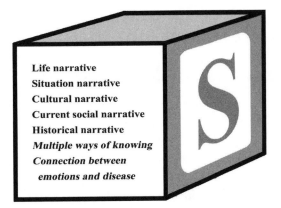

Life narrative
Situation narrative
Cultural narrative
Current social narrative
Historical narrative
Multiple ways of knowing
Connection between emotions and disease

FIGURE 1.10 QUALITIES OF STORIES/NARRATIVE-BASED EVIDENCE.

Biomedical physicians have been exploring the intersection of narrative and scientific evidence for over a decade. Greenhalgh (1999), senior lecturer in the Royal Free and University College, London Medical School, wrote:

> *Clinical method is an interpretive act, which draws on narrative skills to integrate the overlapping stories told by patients, clinicians, and test results. The art of selecting the most appropriate medical maxim for a particular clinical decision is acquired largely through the accumulation of "case expertise" (the stories or "illness scripts" of patients and clinical anecdotes). The dissonance we experience when trying to apply research findings to the clinical encounter often occurs when we abandon the narrative-interpretive paradigm and try to get by on "evidence" alone. (p. 323)*

More recently, nurses have started to challenge the assumption that the only valid evidence is acquired through logical empiricism. Nurse educators Rolfe and Gardner (2005) wrote:

> *Nursing is a series of individual and unique encounters, which cannot be described by a science of large numbers. The resulting "science of the unique" is concerned with persons rather than people, with wet data from the clinical setting rather than dry data from the laboratory and clinical trial, and with the individual practice encounter as the site of reflexive research. In particular, we argue that the traditional concept of evidence from formal research is merely the starting point for the on-the-spot generation of reflective/reflexive evidence by nurses themselves as part of everyday practice. (p. 297)*

NOTE

"Wet data" is related to in vivo studies, or science that observes the whole living organism. "Dry data" on the other hand is related to in vitro studies, or science that observes a part of the organism that has been removed from the whole.

Traditionally, holistic nursing practice included deep valuing of individual, social, and cultural narratives. During the mid to late 20th century, the nursing profession all too often appeared to forget this critical base of knowledge in pursuit of its own science. Potter's 2013 BASE of Nursing recaptures this essential aspect of the nursing paradigm. Stories and narrative-based practice are now a prime target for nursing research, education, and practice.

In short, nursing medicine defines knowledge in a more holistic manner that includes not only evidence from scientific studies but also evidence from the interaction of nurses with patients and their families and from nurses' observations about the patient's environment.

Evidence From Science

The science of nursing is growing exponentially (Figure 1.11). Nurse researchers are involved in studies ranging from genomics to the science of caring. At the same time, research findings are being rapidly translated into practice by a growing number of nurses with their Doctor of Nursing Practice degree. These two areas of scholarship—theory and translation into practice—have firmly established a unique field of nursing knowledge. Nurses are now recognized for practicing science-based medicine similar to other health care specialties.

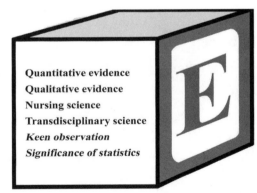

FIGURE 1.11 QUALITIES OF SCIENCE-BASED EVIDENCE.

Much is said about evidence-based nursing practice. However, what started as a movement to ensure greater scientific backing of nursing interventions has turned into the domination of nursing practice by logical empiricism. The nursing paradigm is far more inclusive than this single element and practice, and nursing education depends on mastery of the entire paradigm, not just one domain.

Comparison of Professional Paradigms

Each health care profession has unique domains of knowledge and relationship. But health professions also have overlapping areas of knowledge and shared relationships. Shared areas include knowledge based on the scientific method. Nurses and physicians also share similar ethical values, including non-maleficence and beneficence as principles for relationships. In addition, many nurses and physicians believe that our minds, bodies, and spirits impact both health and illness. And most physicians, nurses, and other health care providers are motivated by care and concern for people.

However, while nursing and biomedicine share particular activities/skills and evidence from research, they also have unique fields of knowing and relating (Figure 1.12).

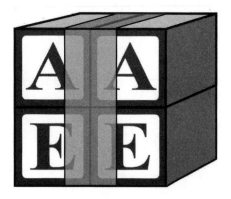

FIGURE 1.12 SHARED AND UNIQUE FIELDS OF KNOWING AND RELATING.

Whereas the unique focus of research for physicians may be the impact a drug has on the physiology of the human body, a nurse researcher may focus her or his research on the management of side effects related to the drug or the knowledge a client needs to be able to adhere to a medication regimen.

The actions of physicians may generally focus on the diagnosis and treatment of conditions impacting health, while nurses' actions include creating environments where patients have the best chance of healing. Nonetheless, nurses and physicians share fields of knowledge and relating. For instance, nurses may use research findings reported in the *New England Journal of Medicine* or *The Lancet* to inform their practice; their nursing research; and education of students, patients, families, and communities. In addition, nurses and physicians share aspects of active caring such as interdependent interventions, advocacy, and patient/family/community education.

The differences between the nursing paradigm and the biomedical paradigm are often subtle. Yet the hierarchical ranking of these two paradigms persists in practice. Indeed, the overlapping fields of knowledge and relationships shared by nurses and physicians have frequently led others to falsely assume nursing is nothing but a medical model with limitations.

Being able to articulate nursing's unique medicine (see Table 1.1) allows nurses to advocate for full and equal partnership in leading health care and is indispensable for nurses to be full partners in interprofessional teams.

TABLE 1.1 Nursing's Unique Medicine

MEDICINE SHARED BY NURSES AND PHYSICIANS	NURSING'S MEDICINE
Care about the patient	Care for the patient, care expands from feeling to action.
	Caring is not limited to skilled interventions. Caring is also demonstrated through skilled use of therapeutic presence.

continues

TABLE 1.1 Continued

MEDICINE SHARED BY NURSES AND PHYSICIANS	NURSING'S MEDICINE
	Nursing's medicine includes caring not only for the patient, but for the family, friends, and community of the patient.
Are concerned about the physical condition of the patient	Nursing's medicine is decidedly holistic. The physical status is only one component of the wellness state. The mind-body-spirit is one totality; therefore, the nurses' focus must be on restoration of the whole integrated system.
Conduct initial assessments that include: • Subjective data: Chief concern, history of present illness, past medical history, family history, social history including risk factors and current lifestyle • Objective data: Head-to-toe assessment or review of systems	Nursing medicine uses subjective and objective data and narrative data. Narrative data may include: • Listening for the story that the patient and family use to talk about the illness or condition. • How do they make meaning of the illness? • Do they blame the illness or condition on a particular event or person? • Do they think it is possible to have improved health? • What are their personal health care goals? • How are the patient and family coping with the situation? • Does anything help them cope? • What are the dominant emotions being experienced by the patient and family at this time?

MEDICINE SHARED BY NURSES AND PHYSICIANS	NURSING'S MEDICINE
	• Is there a cultural story related to the patient's illness or condition (for example, historical trauma experienced by Native Americans or racism experienced by African Americans)?
	• What is the patient and family's previous experience with health care providers? Was it positive? Fear-provoking?
	• Are the patient and family prepared to be full partners in their health care?
Analyze the data: Determine the problem, list potential diagnoses (medical or nursing) causing the acute problem or describe the status of a chronic problem, and support the conclusion with clinical reasoning or evidence	Nursing medicine also includes the patient and family's input into the analysis. Does the analysis "ring true"? Do they want to add additional data that has not been considered? The problems defined may also be systemic in nature, reflecting the holistic approach of nursing medicine.
Perform evidence-based interventions	Nursing medicine uses both evidence-based interventions (generalizable) and interventions designed for each unique individual.
Evaluate responses to interventions and treatments	Because the nurse usually spends significantly more time with a patient, the nurse is generally the first health professional to note the patient's response to prescribed treatments.
Work collaboratively with other health professionals	Encourage collaboration with the patient and family or community
Participate in ongoing professional development to maintain licensure or certification	

continues

TABLE 1.1 Continued

MEDICINE SHARED BY NURSES AND PHYSICIANS	NURSING'S MEDICINE
Participate in professional organizations and conduct and disseminate research to advance knowledge in the profession	
Nurses and physicians both have an orientation toward service, a specialized body of knowledge, practical and theoretical education, autonomy, knowledge based on scientific research, representation by a professional organization, an extended period of education, ongoing professional development, and standards of practice to guide their profession.	The Flexner Report written in 1915 defined modern medical education and practice. The report did not, however, include ethical behavior as a criterion for the medical profession. On the other hand, ethical comportment is a fundamental pillar of professional nursing (Potter, 2010).
Registered nurses and physicians develop a treatment plan, do patient education, and plan for follow-up. Both advanced practice registered nurses and physicians can order diagnostic testing and prescribe pharmaceuticals.	Physicians may prescribe pharmaceuticals or order treatments, but the nurse is generally the one to administer these particular interventions. Nursing medicine dedicates far more time to patient and family education. The education is planned and continuous, and the patient/family is regularly evaluated for degree of understanding and retention, whereas patient education done by physicians is generally spontaneous, episodic, and the patient is rarely evaluated for understanding and retention. When physicians do patient education, families may be present but involvement is frequently minimal.

Nursing's Unique Medicine

The benefits of the unique medicine of nursing are increasingly recognized. An example is this results summary of a recent Gallup survey commissioned by the Robert Wood Johnson Foundation (RWJF, 2010): "From reducing medical errors, to increasing the quality of care, to promoting wellness, to improving efficiency and reducing costs, a new survey finds that an overwhelming majority of opinion leaders say nurses should have more influence" (para. 1).

However, the resistance to this greater influence was also recognized in this same poll: "But these opinion leaders—including insurance, corporate, health services, government and industry thought leaders as well as university faculty— see significant barriers that prevent nurses from fully participating as leaders in health and health care" (para. 1). One barrier has been that nurses themselves have found it difficult to define and defend their unique medicine. This is why the BASE of Nursing needs to be part of nursing education.

As you have seen, while there are overlaps, the medicine of physicians is primarily based on only two domains: active caring and evidence based in science. By contrast, nursing's medicine is primarily based on four domains: being present, active caring, stories/narrative evidence, and evidence based in science. Comparing these two paradigms, you see that *consistently being present* and *consistent* use of *stories or narrative-based evidence* differentiate the medicine of nursing from the medicine of physicians. Of course, there will always be exceptions. A physician may have good "bedside manner," but it is not the expectation. Physicians are expected to be expert diagnosticians and prescribers of effective treatment plans. On the other hand, the nursing profession places great emphasis on, and dedicates more time to, mastery of therapeutic presence and collection of narrative-based evidence.

Nurses use presence and stories to bring healing and wholeness to patients, families, and communities. In these and other ways, the medicine of nursing is deeply connected to partnership.

Conclusion

A partnership approach is the framework for nursing medicine, and partnership allows each domain of the nursing paradigm to reach its full potential. Through partnership, nurses are present to individuals and communities in times of joy as well as times of suffering. Through physical, psychological, emotional, and spiritual presence with individuals, families, and communities, nurses become privy to deep and significant stories of hope and fear. Based on these stories, nurses craft interventions and nurturing environments that allow the restorative processes of the mind, body, and spirit to be activated. That, after all, is the true medicine of nursing.

References

American Nurses Association (ANA). (2007). *Holistic nursing: Scopes and standards of practice.* Silver Spring, MD: American Nurses Association.

American Nurses Association (ANA). (2013). *What is nursing?* Retrieved from http://www.nursingworld.org/EspeciallyForYou/What-is-Nursing.

Benner, P., Sutphen, M., Leonard, V., & Day, L. (2010). *Educating nurses: A call for radical transformation.* San Francisco, CA: Jossey-Bass.

Castledine, G. (2005). Preserving nursing's identity in interdisciplinary working. *British Journal of Nursing, 14*(12), 681.

Cowin, L. (2001). Measuring nurses' self-concept. *Western Journal of Nursing, 23*(3), 313-325.

Cull-Wilby, B. L., & Pepin, J. I. (1987). Towards a coexistence of paradigms in nursing knowledge development. *Journal of Advanced Nursing, 12*(4), 515-521.

Ehrenreich, B., & English, D. (1973). *Witches, midwives, and nurses: A history of women healers.* New York, NY: The Feminist Press.

Eisler, R. (2002). *The power of partnership: Seven relationships that will change your life.* Novato, CA: New World Library.

Fredriksson, L. (1999). Modes of relating in caring conversation: A research synthesis on presence, touch and listening. *Journal of Advanced Nursing, 30*(5), 1167-1176.

Getzendanner, S. (1988). Permanent injunction order against AMA. *JAMA, 259*(1), 81-82.

Greenhalgh, T. (1999). Narrative based medicine: Narrative based medicine in an evidence based world. *BMJ, 318*(7179), 323-325.

Hanks, R. G. (2010). The medical-surgical nurse perspective of advocate role. *Nursing Forum, 45*(2), 97-107.

Heal. Online Etymology Dictionary. (n.d.) Retrieved from http://www.etymonline.com

Institute of Medicine (IOM). (2010). *The future of nursing: Leading change, advancing health.* Washington, DC: National Academies.

International Council of Nurses (ICN). (2010). Definition of nursing. Retrieved from http://www.icn.ch/about-icn/icn-definition-of-nursing/

Loudon, I. (2006). A brief history of homeopathy. *Journal of the Royal Society of Medicine, 99*(12), 607-610.

McMahon, M. A., & Christopher, K. A. (2011). Toward a midrange theory of nursing presence. *Nursing Forum, 46*(2), 71-82.

Potter, T. M. (2010). Reconstructing a new story of nursing: Critical analysis of nursing textbooks using Riane Eisler's partnership paradigm. *Dissertation Abstracts International, 72*(05), 3447086.

Potter, T. M. (2013). *The BASE of nursing.* Unpublished manuscript, School of Nursing, University of Minnesota, United States of America.

Reeves, R. R., & Burke, R. S. (2009). Perception of osteopathic medicine among allopathic physicians in the deep central southern United States. *Journal of the American Osteopathic Association, 109*(6), 318-323.

Robert Wood Johnson Foundation (RWJF). (2010). Groundbreaking new survey finds that diverse opinion leaders say nurses should have more influence on health systems and services. Retrieved from http://www.rwjf.org/pr/product.jsp?id=54488

Rolfe, G., & Gardner, L. (2005). Towards a nursing science of the unique: Evidence, reflexivity, and the study of persons. *Journal of Research in Nursing, 10*(3), 297-310.

Chapter 2
Interprofessional Education and Practice: A Call for Partnership

"Nurses also should be educated with physicians and other health professionals both as students and throughout their careers in lifelong learning opportunities."

–Institute of Medicine (2010)

The interprofessional education and collaborative practice (IPECP) paradigm has been gaining support for several decades. Interprofessional practice moves away from different health professions simply caring for the same patient and toward patient care delivered by teams of different professionals working together for a common goal. With backing from the World Health Organization (WHO) and governments around the globe, early adopters started drafting the principles of interprofessional education (IPE) and interprofessional practice (IPP) in the later part of the 20th century.

Currently, the increasing complexity of health care is making the need for IPECP obvious, and more and more health professionals are joining the call for change. Education and practice are reaching a tipping point and are likely to shift dramatically. Therefore, best-practice nursing education must have a strong interprofessional component. Indeed, interprofessional education and practice will significantly impact the nursing profession in positive ways. For instance, the 2010 Institute of Medicine report, *The Future of Nursing: Leading Change, Advancing Health*, recommends nurses practice to the full extent of their education—an objective that has a better chance of being met with IPE and IPP.

For nurses to participate as full partners in interprofessional practice, the nursing profession needs to become familiar with the core values and competencies of IPECP. In particular, nurse educators should be well versed in these core values and competencies because they will be writing the curricula that prepare future nurses for collaborative practice. Nurses in practice also need to be educated in the IPECP core competencies, as they will be expected to participate as full partners with other health care professionals.

Health Care Complexity and the Need for Interprofessional Education

The exponentially increasing complexity of health care is a global issue that requires changing how health care services are delivered in both developed and developing nations.

Physicians and nurses have worked side by side throughout history. According to Grumbach and Bodenheimer (2004), interprofessional teams existed in the United States as early as 1915 when physicians, social workers, and health educators worked together in outpatient clinics at Massachusetts General Hospital. But despite evidence of intentional collaboration at the turn of the century, interprofessional teamwork did not gain broader acceptance in the United States until the 1970s. That is when students and professionals, in response to increasing complexity, saw the growing need to shift the health care paradigm.

For instance, in 1970, students from different health professions at the University of Minnesota formed an organization called Council for Health Interdisciplinary Participation (CHIP). The University of Minnesota Alumni News (1972) reported, "Working with others outside their specialties, students have grown to appreciate the skills and knowledge each area of the Health Sciences can contribute to total health care delivery" (p. 16).

At an organizational level, the Institute of Medicine (IOM) was an early adopter and promoter of team or collaborative approaches to health care in the United States (1972). More recently, the IOM report brief on *Crossing the Quality Chasm: A New Health System for the 21st Century* (2001) asserted: "Cooperation among clinicians is a priority. Clinicians and institutions should actively collaborate and communicate to ensure an appropriate exchange of information and coordination of care" (p. 4). IOM reports are very influential in shaping health care policy, practice, and education in the United States. Therefore, interprofessional collaboration will likely be a significant aspect of health care in the future.

These examples of IPE and IPP are from the United States, but many nations have had similar developmental underpinnings. Many have their own Centers for IPE, including the United Kingdom, Europe, Canada, Australia, and Scandinavia. In 2008, the first WHO survey was conducted to determine the breadth and depth of IPE in its 193 member states. Over 41 nations indicated some degree of IPE in their countries (Rodger & Hoffman, 2010). Besides the World Health Organization, other global nonprofit organizations are also leading the IPE and IPP movements, including the Centre for the Advancement of Interprofessional Education (CAIPE) in the United Kingdom and the Canadian Interprofessional Health Collaborative (CIHC). In the United States, many universities have started including IPE in their curriculum. Yale, Vanderbilt, the Universities of Colorado, Minnesota, Virginia, Oklahoma, and others are recognizing the importance of ensuring the health profession curriculum addresses the complex needs of today's health care environment.

In 2011, the United States' Health Resources and Services Administration (HRSA) convened a meeting of the Josiah Macy Jr. Foundation, the Robert Wood Johnson Foundation, the ABIM Foundation, and the Interprofessional Education Collaborative (IPEC). The purpose of the meeting was to advance IPE as a critical national initiative (Team-Based Competencies, 2011). In 2012, the Josiah Macy Jr. Foundation, the John A. Hartford Foundation, the Robert Wood Johnson Foundation, and the Gordon and Betty Moore Foundation, in collaboration with HRSA, established the National Coordinating Center for Interprofessional Education and Collaborative Practice (CC-IPECP) at the University of Minnesota (Academic Health Center, 2012). The indications are that significant monetary investment in IPE is supporting a culture shift where interprofessional education and practice will soon be the norm.

In the United States, several state and national government and nonprofit organizations are championing collaborative practice as a way to improve patient outcomes while decreasing health care costs. For example, the Institute for Healthcare Improvement's (IHI, 2013) *Triple Aim Initiative* directly aligns with IPE and IPP objectives. The Triple Aim is IHI's framework for optimizing health system performance. Objectives include the following:

- Improving the patient experience of care (including quality and satisfaction)

- Improving the health of populations

- Reducing the per capita cost of health care (IHI, 2013, para. 1)

Different organizations and health care systems across the nation are starting to collaborate across traditional boundaries to meet the Triple Aim. For instance, the nonprofit Institute for Clinical Systems Improvement (ICSI) brings physicians, medical groups, policymakers, health care consumers, and five Minnesota and Wisconsin health care plans together to collaborate on Triple Aim objectives (ICSI, 2013a, About ICSI section). In 2008, the State of Minnesota passed legislation to establish Health Care Homes, "an approach to primary care in which primary care providers, families and patients work in partnership to improve health outcomes and quality of life for individuals with chronic health conditions and disabilities" (ICSI, 2013b). A primary ICSI focus is development of the Health Care Home model. The Centers for Medicare and Medicaid Services (CMS) has launched Partnership for Patients, the goal being improved "quality, safety and affordability of health care for all Americans" (CMS, n.d.). The program acknowledges that the partnership between health care providers and patients is critical.

These examples demonstrate that health care providers, health plans, consumers, and policymakers all recognize the need for partnership-based health care. Therefore, partnership-based interprofessional education needs to focus on intensive theory and curriculum development so it can fully meet the pressing needs of practice.

CHAMPIONS FOR PARTNERSHIP-BASED HEALTH CARE

Canadian Interprofessional Health Collaborative (CIHC)

Centre for the Advancement of Interprofessional Education (CAIPE)

Creative Health Care Management

Institute for Clinical Systems Improvement (ICSI)

Institute for Patient- and Family-Centered Care (IPFCC)

Interprofessional Education Collaborative (IPEC)

National Center for Interprofessional Practice and Education

Partnership for Patients initiative, Centers for Medicare and Medicaid Services

Society for Participatory Medicine

Interprofessional Education and the Global Shortage of Health Care Professionals

The worldwide shortage of professionals is another major driver of the movement toward partnership-based interprofessional health care. "The World Health Organization [WHO] estimates a shortage of more than four million doctors, nurses, midwives, and others" (WHO, 2006a, p. 11). Bottom line: There simply are not enough health care providers to meet the escalating need for quality health care.

This shortage impacts the entire globe, albeit disproportionately, with the shortage much greater in the developing world. For instance, Africa needs to see a 139% increase in the number of health care workers (HCWs) in order to meet current demands, whereas the Americas need to increase their number of HCWs by 40% (WHO, 2006a, p. 13). But even then, it is not an easy feat to nearly double the number of HCWs required.

The financial investment per country per year to educate enough HCWs to fill the health care provider gap is estimated by WHO (2006a) to range from $1.6 million US to $2 billion US, depending on the population of the country (p. 13). Yet dramatically increasing the required financial investment is unrealistic for most nations. Therefore, it is essential to develop innovative responses to effectively address this acute problem (WHO, 2006b; WHO, 2011). Interprofessional practice based on interprofessional education is such a response.

Since 1978, the WHO has been a key player in the global promotion of IPE and IPP to address both the global HCW shortage and the increasing complexity of health care needs (WHO, 1978). In 1988, the WHO issued its first technical report on teamwork and collaboration in health care (WHO, 1988). Now IPECP has become a significant part of the WHO mission. In fact, the WHO report *Framework for Action on Interprofessional Education and Collaborative Practice* (2010) suggests that IPE needs to become a required element of education for every health professional. And all current literature published by WHO uses the terms interprofessional education and interprofessional practice.

WHO (2010) states, "Interprofessional education occurs when students from two or more professions learn about, from, and with each other to enable effective collaboration and improve health outcomes" (p. 10). The objectives of this type of education are:

- To prepare students in the health professions to be ready to practice in collaborative teams upon graduation

- To optimize the skills of members

- To promote collaboration on case management

- To improve the quality of health services delivered to individuals and communities (WHO, 2010, p. 10)

According to WHO (2010), the goal of interprofessional education is to prepare a *practice-ready workforce*. A practice-ready workforce denotes HCWs who have been interprofessionally educated and enter the workforce ready to participate in collaborative teams. Preparing a practice-ready workforce, therefore, has significant implications for nursing education and curriculum.

In 2010, *The Lancet* commission of international professionals and academic leaders in health care issued a white paper supporting a new vision for education of physicians, nurses, and public health professionals. *Health Professionals for a New Century: Transforming Education to Strengthen Health Systems in an Interdependent World* (Frenk et al., 2010) includes this vision for health care education:

> *All health professionals in all countries should be educated to mobilise [sic] knowledge and to engage in critical reasoning and ethical conduct so that they are competent to participate in patient and population-centered health systems as members of locally responsive and globally connected teams. The ultimate purpose is to assure universal coverage of the high-quality comprehensive services that are essential to advance opportunity for health equity within and between countries. (p. 1924)*

The Lancet commission (Frenk et al., 2010) cites the global HCW shortage and the increasing complexity of care as the major reasons that health care education must be transformed. The paper demonstrates that teamwork can no longer be considered a secondary focus for professionals: It must be recognized as a key component of effective and efficient systems of health care. This paper has significant implications for the education of health professionals. In nursing, all levels of nursing education must emphasize teamwork if the profession expects to be a full partner with other health care providers and be a significant leader of future health care initiatives.

Benefits of an Interprofessional Approach to Education and Practice

The fields of interprofessional education and practice are anchored in scholarship. This scholarship is needed for IPE faculty and IPP practitioners to implement best-practice initiatives.

The *Journal of Interprofessional Care* is the primary resource documenting cutting-edge research and new developments in IPECP. The WHO also continues to lead the IPECP movement through publication of significant IPECP reports. For example, in 2010 the WHO report *Framework for Action on Interprofessional Education and Collaborative Practice* (WHO, 2010) demonstrated that positive attitudes among the professions are connected to positive patient outcomes. The report stated, "By shifting the way health workers think about and interact with one another, the culture of the working environment and attitudes of the workforce will change, improving the working experience of staff and benefiting the community as a whole" (p. 22).

This 2010 WHO report also summarizes research findings that indicate positive patient and provider outcomes related to collaborative practice:

- Collaborative practice can improve:

    —Access to and coordination of health services
    —Appropriate use of specialist clinical resources
    —Health outcomes for people with chronic diseases
    —Patient care and safety

- Collaborative practice can decrease:

    —Total patient complications
    —Length of hospital stay
    —Tension and conflict among caregivers
    —Staff turnover
    —Hospital admissions
    —Clinical error rates
    —Mortality rates

- In community mental health settings, collaborative practice can:

    —Increase patient and career satisfaction
    —Promote greater acceptance of treatment
    —Reduce duration of treatment
    —Reduce cost of care
    —Reduce incidence of suicide
    —Increase treatment for psychiatric disorders
    —Reduce outpatient visits (WHO, 2010, p. 18)

But while research demonstrates that IPP maximizes the strengths and skills of each health professional, allowing them to practice to their full potential (WHO, 2010), it must be noted that more rigorous research and theory development is still required in interprofessional education and collaborative practice.

In a review of literature, Reeves et al. (2009) found only six randomized control studies that evaluated the correlation between IPP and patient outcomes. A more recent review of literature by Abu Rish et al. (2012) analyzes the results of 83 quantitative, qualitative, and mixed-method IPECP studies. This meta-analysis reveals that IPE yields improved understanding of the roles and scopes of different health professions, improved interprofessional communication skills, and overall student satisfaction with IPE activities. Yet despite these positive findings, some researchers also noted many faculty still lack formal preparation to teach IPE curriculum (Abu Rish et al., 2012). This may contribute to the authors noting inconsistencies in IPE curriculum, as well as the way it is taught, evaluated, and reported. Abu-Rish et al.'s (2012) research confirms earlier studies that indicate IPE best practices are still in formation and often lack a cohesive link between theory and practice.

Because at this point the theoretical underpinnings of interprofessional education and collaborative practice are still emerging, IPECP will greatly benefit from a comprehensive new theoretical framework.

Moving Toward a Partnership-Based Theoretical Framework

A new and cohesive theoretical framework for IPECP is essential if it is to achieve its goals. This need is increasingly recognized by both researchers and practitioners—especially from the nursing profession. Without the core value of respect for each other's contributions, the health care professions can stray onto the familiar turf of rigid hierarchies and interprofessional intimidation. Just because the professions collaborate does not mean they are free of domination.

True partnership requires intentional practice solidly anchored in partnership theory. A number of scholars have noted this problem. For example, Craddock, O'Halloran, McPherson, Hean, and Hammick (2013) reviewed IPE curriculum development literature and found universal implementation of a "top-down approach," with classic threads of domination where managers, deans, and senior faculty mandate implementation of IPE by other faculty. In a "top-down approach," faculty often implemented the most expedient approach to curriculum development (Craddock et al., 2013). "Findings suggest that IPE curriculum developers to date have not used educational theory to underpin the design of IPE initiatives. Instead, they are drawing on their 'everyday' or 'common-sense' approaches to implement successful IPE initiatives" (p. 70). An "everyday" approach holds particular danger of perpetuating the old system. If faculties are not learning a new way of thinking about interprofessional relationships, they may unintentionally socialize new health care providers to maintain a hierarchical relationship between the professions.

As Craddock et al. (2013) note, the faculties were not invited to participate in discussions about IPE theories or philosophy. Instead, they received a directive to include IPE content in their courses. The article concludes, "A top-down approach may lead curriculum developers to be so focused on logistics and making it happen rather than stepping back and exploring the theoretical underpinnings of the curricula they design" (p. 71). Curricula without a solid grounding in theory may prevent IPE from reaching its goal.

A partnership approach to IPE theory and curriculum development is designed to avoid these pitfalls. This approach is on the opposite end of the continuum from a top-down approach, and is already being developed in a number of contexts.

IN-2-THEORY is a wonderful example of partnership in the emerging domain of IPECP theory (Hean et al., 2013). From 2007-2009, the UK Economics and Social Research Council sponsored IPECP leaders in their search for theoretical underpinnings. These leaders utilized a CoP approach where "a group of people who share a concern or a passion for something they do, learn how to do it better as they interact regularly" (Hean et al., 2013, p. 88). In this model of theory development, the theory emerges in the midst of interaction or partnership.

Hugh Barr (2013) has done additional IPECP theory development on behalf of the Centre for the Advancement of Interprofessional Education (CAIPE) in the United Kingdom. He summarizes useful theories for framing the learning context in IPECP. One theory he suggests may be beneficial is *organizational theory*, where:

> *Members foster a culture of enquiry within an organization, which is innovative, proactive and capable of a continuous and cyclical process of change reframing information as learning…. They respect each other's differing roles, experience and expertise, and value them as learning assets. They mobilize their collective capacity to respond to learning needs…. [They rely] on double-loop learning, a flexible response which only the coordinated and committed action of a team or organization can produce within a changing environment, in contrast to single-loop learning which is intent on enhancing an individual's position and progress in competition with others. (pp. 6-7)*

Canada has long been a leader in the interprofessional movement. Hall, Weaver, and Grassau (2013), faculty at the University of Ottawa, have been implementing IPE and IPP or interprofessional care (IPC) in an academic palliative care program since 1997. Over the years they have assembled a theoretical toolbox that they believe beneficial for other educators. Hall, Weaver, and Grassau's primary goal for prelicensure HCWs was to help them "build skills/competencies in IPC before they developed strong professional cognitive maps within their professional cultures" (2013, p. 75).

This belief underscores an important fact about paradigms: Once you are committed to one paradigm, it is very difficult to see an alternative paradigm. For example, once you embrace the domination paradigm, it is difficult to unlearn and move toward partnership. That is why it is so critical for IPE to be grounded in principles of partnership from the very first course. Faculty also must value the partnership paradigm and model partnership behavior with their students. As you will see in succeeding chapters, this paradigm shift can be greatly facilitated by an understanding of Eisler's (1987, 2002) partnership paradigm and her cultural transformation theory.

Another source for developing a partnership paradigm for IPE and IPC, as Hall, Weaver, and Grassau (2013) note, are relationship theories. They write:

> If our goal in IPE is to move beyond the rhetoric that we "should all get along," we need to encourage learners to really think about how they build and sustain strong relationships. Centering on relationships and encouraging learners to think about care provision not as patient-based but "relationship-based" requires learners to reflect and re-examine all they have learned and continue to learn about how to be in relationships. (p. 77)

Eisler's theory takes this a step further: It challenges health care providers to rethink *all* of their relationships including relationship with self, patients/clients, colleagues, other professionals, and communities.

Reeves and Hean (2013), two significant leaders in the IPECP theoretical movement, also make this point. They write that the next theoretical frontier will involve pulling sociological theories about our larger cultural contexts into IPE:

> The limited use of sociological perspectives limits our sociopolitical and economic understanding of how important dimensions such as imbalances in power/status, gender and ethnic differences are enacted in daily practice and how they can affect the delivery of effective interprofessional care. Given recent theoretical advances within the field, we remain confident that such challenges will soon begin to be addressed. (p. 2)

This prescient statement sets the stage for two sociological theories examined later in this book: Eisler's cultural transformation (1987, 2002) and caring economics (2007) theories, which address imbalances in power, gender inequities, and the low value traditionally assigned to the work of caring.

Nursing and Interprofessional Education and Practice

The implications of what you have been exploring for nursing are manifold. Nurses have not been considered equal members of health care teams, and it will take concerted action, including changes in the education of nurses as well as other health care professionals, to change this. According to the Executive summary of the IOM report *Health Professions Education: A Bridge to Quality* (Greiner & Knebel, 2003), "All health professionals should be educated to deliver patient-centered care as members of an interdisciplinary team, emphasizing evidence-based practice, quality improvement approaches, and informatics" (p. 3). Yet policy decisions and education for practice have been very slow to align with this goal (Interprofessional Education Collaborative Expert Panel, 2011; National League for Nursing, n.d.).

In a comprehensive review of current nursing fundamental textbooks, Potter (2010) found very little content on collaboration. The texts mentioned the positive impact that collaboration has on patient care outcomes and on positive career satisfaction for nurses, yet none of the textbooks mentioned interprofessional education, interprofessional practice, or competencies for these fields. Without a designated IPE curriculum, nursing students in the United States will fail to graduate as a "practice ready workforce" (WHO, 2010).

As early as 1995, nursing research began to demonstrate that nurses benefit from interprofessional education (Carpenter, 1995a). Carpenter evaluated the impact of an interprofessional education experience for first-year medical students and fourth-year nursing students. Students worked together in pairs or in small groups on collaborative projects. At the end of the program, "Participants reported increased understanding of the knowledge and skills, roles and duties of the other professions" (1995a, p. 265). Carpenter (1995b) also reported that the medical and nursing students in this study had decreased negative stereotypes of one another following their interprofessional education experience.

Fortunately, nursing education is beginning to place a stronger emphasis on collaboration. For example, the American Association of Colleges of Nursing

(AACN), the leading voice for baccalaureate and graduate nursing education in the United States, has incorporated interprofessional collaboration competencies into its baccalaureate, master's, and advanced practice nursing doctorate education essentials (AACN, 2006, 2008, 2011).

Nonetheless, a literature search of the keywords *nursing* and *interprofessional education* yielded few results. Published papers generally fell into two categories: case studies that describe an interprofessional approach to a particular course (Pardue, 2013; Robinson, Erlen, Rubio, Kapoor, & Poloyac, 2013) and the previously mentioned papers citing evidence in favor of IPE. But in most of these papers the authors discussed IPE in general, not the unique nursing response to IPE.

A sign that the relative scarcity of nursing-specific IPE scholarship may be about to change is the newly formed Interprofessional Education Collaborative (IPEC). IPEC is a collaboration of six U.S. national health profession organizations, including nursing, dentistry, medicine, public health, osteopathic medicine, and pharmacy. The AACN is nursing's IPEC representative (AACN, 2012).

IPEC has published *Core Competencies for Interprofessional Collaborative Practice* (2011). This document describes key IPP competencies that must be demonstrated by graduates from all health profession education programs. This is an important development, but competencies are not sufficient for shifting a culture. At the national conference Team-Based Competencies: Building a Shared Foundation for Education and Practice (2011), it was noted that a significant restraining factor to IPE and IPP is the shortage of faculty familiar with interprofessional collaboration and teamwork skills.

Faculties play a significant role in whether students learn how to be partners. Barr (2013) suggested that in order for IPE to be successful, it must be grounded in an awareness of social theory, especially an understanding of the unique socialization patterns for each profession. This echoes the work of Barnsteiner, Disch, Hall, Mayer, and Moore (2007), who wrote:

Interprofessional learning takes place within a context where differences in culture, beliefs, and prior health care experiences among learners of various professions often exist. Exploring the differences and similarities among professional groups as a part of the interprofessional learning process helps learners to build a solid foundation of understanding upon which future health care partnerships can be built. (p. 146)

In a similar vein, D'Amour and Oandasan (2005), on behalf of Health Canada's IPE efforts, wrote that "Interprofessionality requires a paradigm shift, since interprofessional practice has unique characteristics in terms of values, codes of conduct, and ways of working. These characteristics must be elucidated" (p. 9). To promote this paradigm shift, interprofessional scholarship and education must critically examine the historic relationships between the professions from the perspective of the partnership and domination models. (Chapter 3 in this book does just that.) In so doing, it is critical that remnants of domination patterns be exposed and understood, because domination behaviors threaten the success of IPP.

This book provides knowledge and tools so each health profession can challenge antiquated ways in which it still socializes new members—and instead create new socialization methods that prepare members to be full partners.

Moving Beyond Teamwork and Collaboration to Partnership

Language is an important tool in culture change. Despite shared goals, communication and understanding between people is often limited by language. It is therefore important to carefully create an IPECP lexicon so all parties can use a common vocabulary. For example, *collaboration* and *teamwork* are common IPE terms that need further discussion.

Collaboration is more than cooperation and coordination. The World Health Organization (2010) clarifies the difference:

Many health workers believe themselves to be practicing collaboratively, simply because they work together with other health workers. In reality, they may simply be working within a group where each individual has agreed to use their own skills to achieve a common goal. Collaboration, however, is not only about agreement and communication, but about creation and synergy. Collaboration occurs when two or more individuals from different backgrounds with complementary skills interact to create a shared understanding that none had previously possessed or could have come to on their own. (p. 36)

These are important distinctions. Yet, as Grumbach and Bodenheimer (2004) observe, teamwork and collaboration are not sufficient for creating positive outcomes. They write, "While some team members may shine as initiators, clarifiers, or encouragers, others may play negative roles as dominators, blockers, evaders, and recognition seekers" (p. 250). Therefore, interprofessional education needs to be anchored in the partnership paradigm.

Similarly, Eisler (2002) urges caution with the word *collaboration*, stating that those with power often collaborate to keep others controlled and dependent. Even use of the word *team* needs to be scrutinized because teams can use unethical approaches when they believe the "ends justify the means." Eisler has chosen the word *partnership* to describe an alternative pattern of social organization. She writes:

One overarching myth is that partnership is just another term for working together or collaboration. The reality is that a partnership system refers to much more than collaboration. Collaboration is possible in both the partnership and domination systems, but is patterned differently. (Eisler, n.d., para. 1)

Conclusion

As you will see in the chapters that follow, the partnership paradigm provides the theoretical framework necessary for effective interprofessional relationships. By using a partnership approach, interprofessional practice will be able to reach its full potential as the new norm for health care delivery.

References

Abu-Rish, E., Kim, S., Choe, L., Varpio, L., Malik, E. White, A. A.,...Zierler, B. (2012). Current trends in interprofessional education of health sciences students: A literature review. *Journal of Interprofessional Care, 26*(6), 444-451.

Academic Health Center. (2012). *U of M becomes nation's sole coordinating center for interprofessional education and collaborative practice.* Retrieved from http://www.health.umn.edu/healthtalk/2012/09/18/u-of-m-becomes-nations-sole-coordinating-center-for-interprofessional-education-and-collaborative-practice/

Alumni News-University of Minnesota. (October, 1972). CHIP: Student action for total health care. *Alumni News, University of Minnesota,* 14-17.

American Association of Colleges of Nursing (AACN). (2006). *The essentials of doctoral education for advanced nursing practice.* Washington, DC: The American Association of Colleges of Nursing.

American Association of Colleges of Nursing (AACN). (2008). *The essentials of baccalaureate education for professional nursing practice.* Washington, DC: The American Association of Colleges of Nursing.

American Association of Colleges of Nursing (AACN). (2011). *The essentials of master's education in nursing.* Washington, DC: The American Association of Colleges of Nursing.

American Association of Colleges of Nursing (AACN). (February 15, 2012). *AACN advances nursing's role in interprofessional education.* Retrieved from http://www.aacn.nche.edu/news/articles/2012/ipec

Barnsteiner, J. H., Disch, J. M., Hall, M., Mayer, D., & Moore, S. M. (2007). Promoting interprofessional education. *Nursing Outlook, 55*(3), 144-150.

Barr, H. (2013). Toward a theoretical framework for interprofessional education. *Journal of Interprofessional Care, 27*(1), 4-9.

Carpenter, J. (1995a). Interprofessional education for medical and nursing students: Evaluation of a programme. *Medical Education, 29*(4), 265-272.

Carpenter, J. (1995b). Doctors and nurses: Stereotypes and stereotype change in interprofessional education. *Journal of Interprofessional Care, 9*(2), 151-161.

Centers for Medicare and Medicaid Services (CMS). (n.d.). *Welcome to the partnership for patients.* Retrieved from http://partnershipforpatients.cms.gov/

Craddock, D., O'Halloran, C., McPherson, K., Hean, S., & Hammick, M. (2013). A top-down approach impedes the use of theory? Interprofessional educational leaders' approaches to curriculum development and the use of learning theory. *Journal of Interprofessional Care, 27*(1), 65-72.

D'Amour, D., & Oandasan, I. (2005). Interprofessionality as the field of interprofessional practice and interprofessional education: An emerging concept. *Journal of Interprofessional Care, 19*(Supplement 1), 8-20.

Eisler, R. (n.d.). *Myths about partnership.* Retrieved from the Center for Partnership Studies at http://www.partnershipway.org/core-pathways/abcs-of-dominator-and-partnership-relations/two-social-possibilities-the-domination-system-and-the-partnership-system/?searchterm=collaboration

Eisler, R. (1987). *The chalice and the blade: Our history, our future.* San Francisco, CA: HarperCollins.

Eisler, R. (2002). *The power of partnership: Seven relationships that will change your life.* Novato, CA: New World Library.

Eisler, R. (2007). *The real wealth of nations: Creating a caring economics.* San Francisco, CA: Berret-Koehler.

Frenk, J., Chen, L., Bhutta, Z. A., Cohen, J., Crisp, N., Evans, T.,...Zurayk, H. (November, 2010). Health professionals for a new century: Transforming education to strengthen health systems in an interdependent world. *The Lancet, 376*(9756), 1923-1958.

Greiner, A. C., & Knebel, E. (Eds.). (2003). Health professions education: A bridge to quality (Executive summary). Washington, DC: National Academies.

Grumbach, K., & Bodenheimer, T. (2004). Can health care teams improve primary care practice? *JAMA, 291*(10), 1246-1251.

Hall, P., Weaver, L., & Grassau, P. A. (2013). Theories, relationships and interprofessionalism: Learning to weave. *Journal of Interprofessional Care, 27*(1), 73-80.

Hean, S., Anderson, E., Bainbridge, L., Clark, P. G., Craddock, D., Doucet, S.,... Oandasan, I. (2013). IN-2-THEORY—Interprofessional theory, scholarship and collaboration: A community of practice. *Journal of Interprofessional Care, 27*(1), 88-90.

Institute for Clinical Systems Improvement (ICSI). (2013a). *About ICSI: Who we are.* Retrieved from https://www.icsi.org/about_icsi/

Institute for Clinical Systems Improvement (ICSI). (2013b). *ICSI health care home initiative.* Retrieved from https://www.icsi.org/_asset/03dhmk/health_care_home_summary.pdf

Institute for Healthcare Improvement (IHI). (2013). *IHI Triple Aim Initiative.* Retrieved from http://www.ihi.org/offerings/Initiatives/TripleAim/Pages/default.aspx

Institute of Medicine (IOM). (1972). *Educating for the health team.* (Conference report, October, 1972). Washington, DC: National Academies.

Institute of Medicine (IOM). (2001). *Crossing the quality chasm: A new health system for the 21st century.* (Report brief). Washington, DC: National Academies.

Institute of Medicine (IOM). (2010). *The future of nursing: Leading change, advancing health.* (Report brief). Washington, DC: National Academies.

Interprofessional Education Collaborative Expert Panel. (2011). *Core competencies for interprofessional collaborative practice: Report of an expert panel.* Washington, DC: Interprofessional Education Collaborative.

National League for Nursing. (n.d.). *A nursing perspective on simulation and interprofessional education (IPE): A report from the National League for Nursing's Think Tank on using simulation as an enabling strategy for IPE.* Retrieved from www.nln.org

Pardue, K. T. (2013). Not left to chance: Introducing an undergraduate interprofessional education curriculum. *Journal of Interprofessional Care, 27*(1), 98-100.

Potter, T. M. (2010). Reconstructing a new story of nursing: Critical analysis of nursing text-books using Riane Eisler's partnership paradigm. *Dissertation Abstracts International, 72*(05), 3447086.

Reeves, S., & Hean, S. (2013). Why we need theory to help us better understand the nature of interprofessional education, practice and care. *Journal of Interprofessional Care, 27*(1), 1-3.

Reeves, S., Zwarenstein, M., Goldman, J., Barr, H., Freeth, D., Hammick, M., & Koppel, I. (2009). Interprofessional education: Effects on professional practice and health care outcomes. (Review). *The Cochrane Library,* Issue 4, 2009. Chinchester, UK: Wiley.

Robinson, G. F., Erlen, J. A., Rubio, D. M., Kapoor, W. N., & Poloyac, S. M. (2013). Development, implementation, and evaluation of an interprofessional course in translational research. *Clinical and Translational Science 6*(1), 50-56.

Rodger, S., & Hoffman, S. J. (2010). Where in the world is interprofessional education? A global environment scan. *Journal of Interprofessional Care, 24*(5), 479-491.

Team-Based Competencies. (2011, February). *Team-based competencies: Building a shared foundation for education and clinical practice.* Conference proceedings: Washington, DC.

World Health Organization (WHO). (1978). *Primary health care. Report of the international conference on primary health care.* September 1978. Alma-Ata, USSR. Geneva: World Health Organization.

World Health Organization (WHO). (1988). *Learning together to work together for health.* Report of a WHO study group on multiprofessional education for health personnel: The team approach. Technical Report Series 769: 1-72. Geneva: World Health Organization.

World Health Organization (WHO). (2006a). Health workers: A global profile. *The World Health Report 2006.* Geneva, Switzerland: WHO Press.

World Health Organization (WHO). (2006b). *Taking stock: Task shifting to tackle health worker shortages.* Geneva, Switzerland: WHO Press.

World Health Organization (WHO). (2010). *Framework for action on interprofessional education and collaborative practice.* WHO Department of Human Resources for Health. Geneva, Switzerland: WHO Press.

World Health Organization (WHO). (2011). *Transformative scale up of health professional education: An effort to increase the number of health professionals and to strengthen their impact on population health.* Geneva, Switzerland: WHO Press.

Part II
Reconstructing a Partnership-Based Cultural Narrative

"To dominate socialization means to influence dramatically how people see the world and act on it."
 —*Ira Shor in* Empowering Education:
Critical Teaching for Social Change, *1992, p. 116*

Part II deconstructs the cultural narrative we have been socialized to think of as normal. Deconstructing is an essential prelude to reconstructing both our narratives and our social systems, including our health care systems. As important as it is to create new models, if the old dysfunctional models are not identified and dismantled, they will thwart even the best of new initiatives.

Chapter 3 describes Riane Eisler's cultural transformation theory. The chapter identifies patterns of domination and of partnership in cultures throughout history, as well as foundations for both a more just, caring society and a more effective, inclusive health care system.

Chapter 4 describes Potter's use of Eisler's cultural transformation theory to reexamine the history of nursing. The chapter looks at nursing fundamental textbooks and shows how these have all too often served to perpetuate the domination narrative, with little or no opportunity for students to be exposed to an alternative view or model of nursing. The chapter then tells the first part of a new story of nursing, going back to its earliest roots, which displays more partnership.

Chapter 5 tells the second part of the new story of nursing. For this part of the narrative, Potter uses autobiographies of historic nurses who chose an alternative to domination.

These three chapters socialize nurses to a stronger, more autonomous self-identity, equipping them to be full partners with other professionals.

Chapter 3
Cultural Transformation Theory: A Framework for Nursing Transformation

"The way we structure the most fundamental of all human relations...has a profound effect on every one of our institutions, on our values, and...on the direction of our cultural evolution."
— *Riane Eisler,* The Chalice and the Blade, *1987, p. xix*

In the preceding two chapters, you saw that partnership between the professions is required for successful interprofessional education and practice. You also saw that real partnership is more than just working together or collaboration.

People can, and do, collaborate in systems where one person or group dominates the others. Indeed, people have often collaborated in maintaining their own subordination. Just think of how during the American Civil War some African American house slaves fought on the Southern side to preserve their owners' right to have slaves—including themselves. Even today some women collaborate to maintain their own subordination to men—for example, some Iranian women recently opposed a woman being a judge on the grounds that women are too emotional. The wife of Iran's ambassador to France went so far as to say in an interview with Radio France, "There is a gland in women's heads which makes us emotional, and no matter how powerful we are, this prevents us in critical situations from making the right decisions" (Iran Human Rights Documentation Center, 2013). Or, closer to home, consider how nurses have all too often collaborated in the subordination of their predominantly female profession to that of primarily male physicians.

Fear, be it conscious or unconscious, is one reason for all this collusion by people in their own subordination. Habit, too, has played a part. But a major reason subordinate groups have cooperated in maintaining their inferior status is that they have long been taught that these rankings of domination are inevitable, even moral. For example, when nurses bring a concern to a physician and start the conversation with "I know I am just a nurse but...," this self-subordination causes further disempowerment.

The good news is that there is growing awareness that dominating or being dominated are not our only alternatives. Many people are becoming conscious that relations based on mutual respect, accountability, and caring are possible—indeed—essential if we are to move forward. This awareness is why we hear so much today of the urgent need for cultural transformation, for a fundamental paradigm shift, and with this, a shift in basic beliefs, assumptions, behaviors, and social structures.

This need for a paradigm shift is not only increasingly recognized in the field of health care, but by people and organizations worldwide concerned about meeting our unprecedented economic, environmental, and social challenges. The reason for this focus on a fundamental paradigm shift, as Einstein famously noted, is that we cannot solve problems with the same thinking that created them (thinkexist.com, n.d.).

But what specific changes in beliefs, values, and social structures does a new paradigm require? This question was the impetus for the multidisciplinary, cross-cultural, historical research conducted over several decades by Riane Eisler, one of the authors of this book.

In the introduction to this book, Eisler relates how for her this is not just an academic issue, but one deeply rooted in her early life; as a small child, she and her parents had to flee her native Vienna to escape from the Holocaust. As she also relates, these traumatic experiences led her to questions about human possibilities—questions that eventually led her to reexamine human history and societies.

The Study of Relational Dynamics

As Eisler embarked on her analysis of human societies, she developed the *study of relational dynamics*. This method of inquiry differs markedly from traditional studies of society. Relational dynamics focus on *relationships,* especially:

- What kinds of relationships a particular culture supports or inhibits

- How the key elements of a social system relate to one another to maintain and regenerate the system's basic character (Eisler, 1987, 1993, 1995, 1997, 2003)

The study of relational dynamics draws from a much wider database than that of conventional studies of society. Unlike these studies, which focus primarily on politics and economics, the relational dynamics method of inquiry takes into account the *whole* of peoples' lives—including family and other intimate relations. Unlike the majority of studies, often aptly called "the study of man," relational dynamics takes into account the *whole* of humanity—both its female and male halves. And rather than examining one period at a time, it looks at the *whole* span of history—including the long period before written records called prehistory.

A basic principle of systems theory is that if we do not look at the *whole* of a system, we cannot see the connections between its various components, and thus the system's configuration—just as if we look at only part of a picture, we cannot see the whole picture's configuration. Drawing from a more complete database, the study of relational dynamics makes it possible to see social configurations: connections between different parts of social systems that are not visible through the lenses of conventional social categories such as ancient/modern, Eastern/ Western, religious/secular, rightist/leftist, technologically developed/undeveloped, or capitalist/communist.

Religious/secular, Eastern/Western, and ancient/modern are shorthand for ideological, geographic, and time differences. Right/left and liberal/conservative describe political orientations. Industrial, preindustrial, and postindustrial describe levels of technological development. Capitalism and communism are labels for different economic systems. Democratic/authoritarian describe political systems in which there are, or are not, elections.

Each of these categories leaves out huge swathes of social relations. And all these conventional social categories fail to take into account the importance of the cultural construction of the primary human relations: the formative parent-child relations and the relations between the male and female halves of humanity—even though these relations are basic to our species' survival and to what children learn to view as normal or abnormal, possible or impossible, moral or immoral. In other words, these categories leave out information that is essential if we are to understand why people learn to view human rights violations as acceptable and even moral, or alternately, learn respect for human rights.

Because the quality of the relations a child experiences and observes plays a critical role in the development of nothing less than the human brain, we need categories that take into account the cultural construction of parent-child relations. Because we are a dimorphic species (that is, one consisting of two basic forms), we need classifications that take into account the cultural construction of the roles and relations of the female and male halves of humanity. Because people spend most of their lives in the day-to-day relations of family, school, and local community, we need categories that include what happens in the private spheres as well as the larger public political and economic spheres. And because our problems—personal, political, economic, and ecological—revolve around how we relate to ourselves, others, and the Earth, we need social categories that show what kinds of relations a culture supports or inhibits, be it in families or in the family of nations.

Using the larger database described earlier in this chapter, Eisler (1987) searched for patterns or social configurations that take the above factors into account. What became apparent were configurations that repeat themselves cross-culturally and historically—social configurations that are not visible through the fragmenting lenses of old social categories.

There were no names for these social configurations, so she called one the *domination model* and the other the *partnership model*. No society orients completely to either the domination model or the partnership model. Rather, societies fall on a *partnership/domination continuum*. And the degree to which a society's families, education, religion, politics, economics, and other institutions orient to either end of this continuum profoundly affects everything—including health care.

The Domination and the Partnership Configurations

The domination model and the partnership model have very different social configurations that can be recognized by their core, mutually supporting components (see Figure 3.1).

The Partnership System

Democratic and economically equitable structure

Mutual respect and trust with low degree of violence

Equal valuing of males and females and high regard for stereotypical feminine values

Beliefs and stories that give high value to empathic and caring relations

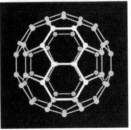

The Domination System

Authoritarian and inequitable social and economic structure

High degree of abuse and violence

Subordination of women and "femininity" to men and "masculinity"

Beliefs and stories that justify and idealize domination and violence

FIGURE 3.1 THE PARTNERSHIP AND DOMINATION SYSTEMS.

Reprinted from Riane Eisler (2007) The Real Wealth of Nations: Creating a Caring Economy *(San Francisco, CA: Berrett-Koehler)*

The Domination Configuration Core Components

The domination configuration comprises these four core components.

- The first core component of the domination configuration is a structure of rigid top-down rankings: hierarchies of domination maintained through physical, psychological, and economic control. This structure is found in both the family and the state or tribe, and is the template for all social institutions. This is the template we have inherited for our health care system, where the doctor "gives orders" that both nurses and patients are expected to obey.

- The second core component of domination systems is the rigid ranking of one half of humanity over the other half. Theoretically, this could be the female half over the male half, but historically, it has been the ranking of the male half over the female half. Once again, we have inherited this ranking of male over female in our health care system, and this ranking is a major obstacle to effective interprofessional education and practice.

- The third core component of the domination model is culturally accepted abuse and violence—ranging from child and wife beatings and abuse of "inferiors" (such as people who are physically, mentally, or emotionally challenged), violence against nonconformists and others who are different, as well as to pogroms, lynchings, and chronic warfare. Every society has some abuse and violence. But in cultures orienting to the domination model, we find the institutionalization and even idealization of abuse and violence to maintain hierarchies of domination—man over woman, man over man, race over race, religion over religion, tribe over tribe, nation over nation, and so on. Today, abuse and violence against people who are physically, mentally, or emotionally challenged is no longer accepted practice, but abuse and violence are still found in some health care systems.

- The fourth core component of the domination model consists of beliefs that relations of domination and submission (beginning with the domination of male over female) are inevitable, normal, and even moral, and that both war and the "war of the sexes" are inevitable. Though many health care providers today reject this belief system on the conscious level, it often maintains its unconscious hold and is still the norm in some cultures and subcultures.

As we will discuss later in this chapter, much of modern history has consisted of challenges to entrenched traditions of domination. However, you can clearly see the domination configuration when looking at some of the most brutally violent and repressive societies of modern times: Hitler's Germany (a technologically advanced, Western, rightist society); Stalin's USSR (a secular leftist society); Khomeini's Iran (an Eastern religious society); and Idi Amin's Uganda (a tribalistic society). Viewed through the lenses of conventional social categories, these seem like completely different societies. But they all share the core configuration of the domination system:

- Authoritarian rule in both the family and state

- The rigid ranking of the male half of humanity over the female half

- A high degree of socially accepted, even idealized, violence

- Beliefs and stories that present all this as normal, even moral

The Partnership Configuration

The partnership model has a very different core configuration. The basic template of this model also consists of four interactive, mutually supporting components.

- The first core component is a democratic and egalitarian structure. This structure is found in both the family and the state or tribe, and is the template for other institutions. That is not to say that no rankings exist. However, these rankings are what Eisler calls *hierarchies of actualization* rather than *hierarchies of domination*. Hierarchies of actualization are more flexible; power is viewed not as power *over* but as power *to* and power *with*. This is the kind of power described in some of today's progressive management literature as empowering rather than disempowering, as inspiring and supporting rather than controlling (Conger & Kanungo, 1988; Eisler, 2007). We will have more to say about these hierarchies of actualization in Chapter 10 when we explore how the partnership model offers a framework for nursing transformation and effective interprofessional education and practice.

- The second core component of partnership systems is equal partnership between women and men, as well as a high valuing, in *both* women and men, of qualities and behaviors such as nonviolence, nurturance, and caregiving—qualities denigrated as "soft," "feminine," and "unmanly" in the domination model. As we will also examine later in this book, this component of partnership systems is of particular relevance to interprofessional education and practice—and to a more caring and effective health care system.

- The third core component of the partnership model is that abuse and violence is not culturally accepted. This does not mean that no abuse or violence are present. But abuse or violence does not have to be institutionalized or idealized because it is not needed to maintain rigid rankings of domination. We will also look at this component of partnership systems later in this book in relation to a more effective and caring health care system.

- The fourth core component of the partnership model consists of beliefs about human nature that support empathic and mutually respectful relations. Although insensitivity, cruelty, and violence are recognized as human possibilities, they are not considered inevitable and normal, much less moral. Again, we will look at the importance of beliefs and stories as they relate to the future of nursing, especially when we examine what stories are still told—and what stories need to be told—about nursing in both popular culture and the education of nurses (Chapters 4 and 6).

Societies that lean toward the partnership end of the continuum also transcend conventional categories such as religious or secular, Eastern or Western, industrial, preindustrial, postindustrial, and so on. For example, the Teduray forest people of the Philippines, as University of California anthropologist Stuart Schlegel observed, can best be described as a partnership society: "I used to call them 'radically egalitarian," Schlegel writes, "But... they have the core configuration characteristic of the partnership model: they are generally egalitarian, women and men have equal status, and they are peaceful"

(1998, p. 244). In describing his fieldwork among the Teduray, Schlegel further writes: "Softer, stereotypically 'feminine' virtues were valued; and community well-being was the principal motivation for work and other activities. Nature and the human body were given great respect. The emphasis on technology was on enhancing and sustaining life" (p. 244).

The agrarian Minangkabau also orient to the partnership model. The Minangkabau are the fourth largest ethnic group in the Sumatran archipelago, numbering about 4 million people (Sanday, 2002). As among the Teduray, here women play major social roles, violence is not part of Minangkabau child rearing, and stereotypically feminine values such as caring and nurturing are valued in both women and men.

In contrast to more domination-oriented ideologies, in the Minangkabau belief system nurture is a basic principle of nature. As University of Pennsylvania anthropologist Peggy Sanday (2002) reports:

The Minangkabau weave order out of their version of wild nature by appeal to maternal archetypes. Unlike Darwin in the 19th century, the Minangkabau subordinate male dominion and competition, which we consider basic to human social ordering and evolution, to the work of maternal nurture, which they hold to be necessary for the common good and the healthy society…Social well-being is found in natural growth and fertility according to the dictum that the unfurling, blooming, and growth in nature is our teacher. (pp. 22-24)

Over the last several centuries, especially in technologically developed, industrialized Western countries, there has been movement toward the partnership end of the continuum. This orientation to the partnership configuration is today most clearly visible in Nordic societies, such as Sweden, Finland, Iceland, and Norway. See Table 3.1.

These Nordic nations are not utopian, but they have more democracy in both the family and the state; suffer no huge gaps between haves and have-nots; view women and men as equals; consider nurturance and nonviolence appropriate behavior for men as well as women; and, support caring and nonviolence in their national policies. For example, they have universal health care, high-quality early childhood education, stipends to help families care for children, and generous paid parental leave for both mothers and fathers. They also pioneered the world's first peace studies programs and the first legislation that makes physical discipline of children in families against the law (Eisler, 2007).

TABLE 3.1 Comparison of the Domination and Partnership Systems

COMPONENT	DOMINATION SYSTEM	PARTNERSHIP SYSTEM
1. Structure	Authoritarian structure of ranking and hierarchies of domination in both family and state or tribe.	Democratic structure of linking and hierarchies of actualization in both family and state or tribe.
2. Gender	Ranking of the male half of humanity over the female half, as well as rigid gender stereotypes, with traits and activities viewed as masculine ("toughness" and conquest) ranked over those seen as feminine ("softness" and caregiving).	Equal valuing of the male and female halves of humanity, as well as fluid gender roles with a high valuing of empathy, caring, caregiving, and nonviolence in both women and men, as well as in social and economic policy.
3. Relations	High degree of fear, abuse, and violence ranging from child and wife beating to other forms of abuse by "superiors" in families, workplaces, and society. Children grow up in punitive, authoritarian, male-dominated families where they observe and experience inequality and inequity as the accepted norm.	Mutual respect and trust with a low degree of fear, abuse, and violence, since they are not required to maintain rigid rankings of domination. Children grow up in families where parenting is authoritative rather than authoritarian and adult relations are egalitarian and equitable.
4. Beliefs	Beliefs and stories that justify and idealize domination and violence, which are presented as inevitable, moral, and desirable.	Beliefs and stories that give high value to empathic, mutually beneficial, non-violent relations, which are considered moral and desirable.

Cultural Transformation Theory

Before turning to the implications of the partnership configuration for a more caring and effective health care system, here we want to briefly outline Eisler's (1987) *cultural transformation theory* and the light it sheds on the paradigm shift needed for successful interprofessional education and practice.

Cultural transformation theory proposes that the tension between the partnership and domination models as two basic ways of structuring institutions, beliefs, and behaviors underlies cultural evolution. It further proposes that by examining this tension, we can better predict the outcome of different personal and cultural choices and thus more effectively intervene in our individual and collective futures (Eisler, 1987, 1995, 1997, 2000, 2002, 2003).

Cultural transformation theory is part of a whole constellation of new theories, including systems theory, cybernetics, chaos theory, evolutionary and complexity theories, as well as nonlinear dynamics (Maturana & Varela, 1980; Prigogine & Stengers, 1984). While it draws from these theories and parallels them, it also expands them by focusing on matters that are not included in them.

Cultural transformation theory draws from other new scholarly strands, including gender and women's and men's studies. In addition, it draws from both recent and early research in biological and social science in its focus on the interaction between biology and culture and among genes, cultures, and individual beliefs and behaviors. But cultural transformation theory provides a new connectivity to some of the insights advanced by other scholars by offering the new, more inclusive conceptual framework of the partnership/domination continuum.

One of the premises of cultural transformation theory is that biology must be considered when studying humanity. This idea is certainly not new; it goes back to Charles Darwin and even earlier evolutionary thinkers. The premise that culture plays a major role in how humans view and live in the world is also not new. It is the basis of sociology and anthropology.

Also not new is the idea, key to cultural transformation theory, that early childhood experiences profoundly affect how we see the world and live in it. This is an insight widely discussed and documented in the psychological literature and the more recent work of neuroscientists such as Bruce Perry, Debra Niehoff, Steven Quartz, and Terrence Sejnowski verify this connection on a biological level (Niehoff, 1999; Perry, n.d.; Quartz & Sejnowski, 2002). However, cultural transformation theory takes this knowledge beyond its usual focus on individual and family dynamics and integrates it into the study of society.

The tenet that the social construction of the roles and relations of women and men is a key component of culture is also not new. This has been documented by many feminist scholars, from Charlotte Perkins Gilman (2007) to bell hooks (1984) and Linda Kerber and Jane De Hart Mathews (1982). Anthropologists such as Peggy Sanday (2002) and Stuart Schlegel (1998) and cultural historians such as Renate Bridenthal and Claudia Koonz (1977) have focused on the connection between culture and the status of women. But cultural transformation theory brings these insights into a more inclusive and integrated explanatory whole that fully takes into account principles of *self-organization* (how systems maintain themselves) and *systems transformation* (how systems are transformed at critical points).

FURTHER READINGS ON GENDER STUDIES

Here is a sampling of some basic books and articles from the relatively new fields of women's studies and men's studies for readers who want to go deeper:

Bernard, J. (1981). The Female World. *New York: Free Press.*

Brod, H. (1987). The Making of Masculinities: The New Men's Studies. *Boston: Allen & Unwin.*

Collins, P. H. (1991). Black Feminist Thought. *New York: Routledge.*

Eisler, R. (1978). The Equal Rights Handbook: What ERA Means to Your Life, Your Rights, and the Future. *New York: Avon Books.*

Eisler, R. (1987). *Human Rights: Toward an Integrated Theory for Action.* The Human Rights Quarterly, 9(3), 287-308.

Fiorenza, E. S. (1983). In Memory of Her. *New York: Crossroads.*

Flexner, E. (1959). Century of Struggle: The Woman's Rights Movement in the United States. *Cambridge, MA: Harvard University Press.*

Gilligan, C. (1982). In a Different Voice. *Cambridge, MA: Harvard University Press.*

Kivel, P. (1992). Men's Work: How to Stop the Violence That Tears Our Lives Apart. *New York: Ballantine Books.*

Martin, E. (1991). The Egg and the Sperm: How Science Has Constructed a Romance Based on Stereotypical Male-Female Roles. Signs, 16(3), 485-501.

Miedzian, M. (1991). Boys Will Be Boys. *New York: Anchor Books.*

Millett, K. (1970). Sexual Politics. *New York: Doubleday.*

Smith, J. (1989). Misogynies. *New York: Fawcett Columbine.*

Spender, D., ed. (1983). Feminist Theorists: Three Centuries of Key Women Thinkers. *New York: Pantheon Books.*

Zihlman, A. (1989). Common Ancestors and Uncommon Apes. In John R. Durant (Ed.). Human Origins *(pp. 81-105). Oxford: Clarendon Press.*

Sample Fiction:

Chopin, K. 1972 (originally published in the 19th century). The Awakening. *New York: Avon Books.—A pathbreaking short story about a 19th-century woman who defies convention.*

Franklin, M. (1980). My Brilliant Career. *New York: St. Martin Press.—A tongue in cheek semi-autobiography written when the author was 18, also made into a good film.*

Hosseini, K. (2008). A Thousand Splendid Suns. *New York: Riverhead.— The moving tale about women in Afghanistan by a sensitive man.*

Rhys, J. (1998). Wide Sargasso Sea. *New York: Norton.—A brilliant retelling of the famous novel Jane Eyre from the perspective of the wife locked up in the attic. The film version does not do this book justice.*

Cultural transformation theory posits that in studying social institutions and human behaviors, we have to take into account the interaction between genes and experiences as influenced by our environments—and that the most important environments for humans at this point in our evolution are our cultural environments. In other words, our human experiences are largely molded by our cultures.

The issue is what *conditions* lead to the expression or inhibition of different aspects of our large and varied human biological repertoire. Even more specifically, the issue is what conditions lead to the expression or inhibition of our great human capacity for empathy, caring, and creativity—or, alternately, for insensitivity, cruelty, and destructiveness (de Waal, 2009; Eisler, 1987, 1995, 2000, 2002). Effectively addressing this issue requires particular focus on the cultural construction of the primary human relations: the relations between women and men and between parents and children that provide our first mental and, as neuroscience now shows, neural) templates for human relations (Perry, n.d.; Quartz & Sejnowski, 2002).

Cultural transformation theory further proposes that human cultural evolution has not been, as we are often taught, a linear progression from "primitive" to "civilized." Instead of a conceptual framework that is unilinear, it offers one that is multilinear (Eisler, 1987, 1993, 1995, 1997, 2000, 2002).

Borrowing a term from the study of nonlinear dynamics, cultural transformation theory proposes that the partnership model and the domination model are two basic *attractors* for social systems. It also proposes that movement from one model to the other does *not* follow a linear progression, and that times of disequilibrium—such as the current one—offer the opportunity for fundamental cultural transformation.

Change is, of course, a constant in the living world. But there is a big difference between change within the parameters of a particular social system and transformative change. The first kind of change does not alter a social system's basic identity or configuration. The second kind of change shifts the system from one basic identity or configuration to another.

Transformative change is the focus both of cultural transformation theory and of those who recognize we must go beyond surface changes to build a system of health care based on principles of partnership.

The Early Direction of Culture

In *The Chalice and the Blade: Our History, Our Future* (Eisler, 1987) and other books, Eisler details findings from archeology, mythology, and other disciplines that suggest that many of our current problems are rooted in a massive cultural transformation in prehistory. These books describe evidence that the original direction of culture, going back to the Old Stone Age or Paleolithic, oriented more toward the partnership model.

To begin with, the art of this period indicates that the powers that govern the universe were not imaged in the form of male deities that have the power to take life, such as Zeus with his sword or Jehovah with his thunderbolt. Rather, they were imaged more in terms of the power to give and nurture life in a nature-based spirituality. To illustrate, the 30,000-year-old Stone Age representations of the nude female body that 19th-century archaeologists called "Venuses" are recognized by Alexander Marshack (1991), James Mellaart (1967), Marija Gimbutas (1982), and other scholars as some of the first Western religious goddess figures. With their prominent breasts, hips, and vulvas, these figures—emphasizing woman's life-giving and nurturing powers—seem to have been part of a mythology focused on nature's cycles of life, death, and regeneration.

Eisler notes that some archeologists still insist that these female images had no religious significance—even though we know that most ancient art was of a religious or spiritual nature, like most art until recent times. They even claim that these works of art were just dolls—despite the fact that some of them are carved into walls of caves or cave entrances, and, not being portable, cannot be dolls.

A striking example is the remarkable stone carving of a nude female figure known as the Venus of Laussal (Figure 3.2), carved about 25,000 years ago at the entrance of a French cave-sanctuary (Eisler, 1987). In one hand, the figure in this carving holds a crescent moon with 13 notches (the number of the cycles of the moon as well as of woman's menstrual cycles). Her other hand points to a sharply etched vulva, indicating that this cave was probably the site of ancient rituals connected with woman's capacity to give life, as represented by her monthly bleeding.

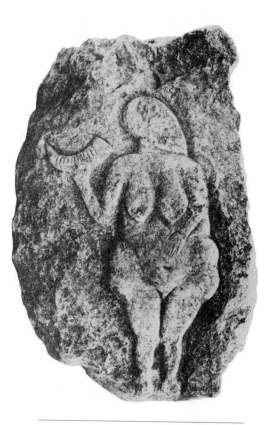

FIGURE 3.2 VENUS OF LAUSSEL.

Another noteworthy aspect of our more partnership-oriented prehistory is represented in images of giving birth found as part of sacred imagery. For example, in the later Neolithic site of Çatalhoyük in Turkey, an 8,000-year-old figure of a seated goddess (see Figure 3.3) is giving birth (Mellaart, 1967).

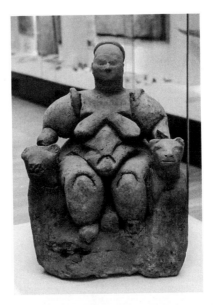

FIGURE 3.3 ÇATALHOYÜK GODDESS GIVING BIRTH.
(Source: Archiwum "Roweromaniaka wielkopolskiego" No_B19-36)

These images starkly contrast with the sacred imagery from later times that oriented much more closely to the domination model. Consider the images of Zeus, Ares, Thor, and other martial deities; of a punitive all-powerful God or Lord in Judeo-Christian-Muslim tradition; or of armed deities chopping one another to death in the Hindu Mahabarata (see Figure 3.4).

The focus on the power to give life and pleasure, rather than on inflicting pain and causing death, is also illustrated by Paleolithic images of vulvas and phalluses. Some archeologists have regarded these as obscene or simply ignored them (Eisler, 1995), but French archeologist André Leroi-Gourhan (1971) points out that these sexual images signal that people of that era were aware that life is renewed through the union of female and male. These images, like the fact that many cave paintings of animals are of pairs of females and males (see Figure 3.5), are expressions of a belief system focusing on the regeneration of life.

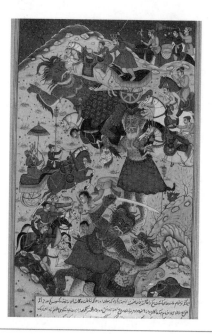

FIGURE 3.4 BATTLE SCENE FROM THE MAHABARATA.

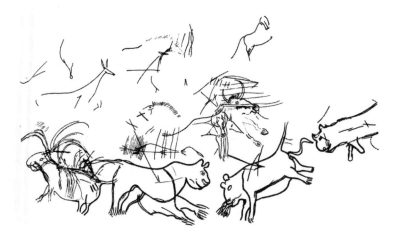

FIGURE 3.5   CAVE PAINTING OF ANIMALS IN PAIRS.

The Next Eras in Cultural Evolution

This theme of the connection between sex and the regeneration of life continues into the Neolithic era (the first Western agrarian civilizations that began about 10,000 years ago). Indeed, it is here that you find the first sculptures of female and male union. One example is the 8,000-year-old sculpture of the so-called *Gumelnita lovers*, excavated near Casciorele in the East Balkans (Gimbutas, 1982). Another is the remarkable stone plaque of a woman and man embracing each other, followed by the woman holding a baby in her arms, excavated in the Neolithic site of Çatal Hüyük (Mellaart, 1967). This plaque seems to depict the observation that both human and animal mating is followed by the birth of offspring. And, like the Gumelnita lovers, this work of art also seems to be a precursor of what scholars later came to call the *hieros gamos* or sacred union (Eisler, 1995).

This sacred union is also a theme in the first writings of Western civilization—the cuneiform tablets of the ancient civilization of Sumer. A notable example is the *Hymns of Inanna*, which celebrate the sacred union of Inanna, the Sumerian Queen of Heaven and Earth, and her lover, the king-god Dumuzi (see Figure 3.6). These ancient writings reveal that not only the return of life, but also the celebration of love and pleasure were central to this ancient belief system.

In passages combining sexual imagery with images of the earth's fecund beauty, Inanna's breasts are described as pouring out plants and water. Wolkstein and Kramer (1983) quote other passages dealing with sensual pleasure and love:

> *He put his hand in her hand.*
> *He put his hand to her heart.*
> *Sweet is the sleep of hand-to-hand.*
> *Sweeter still the sleep of heart-to-heart.*
> *(Wolkstein & Kramer, 1983)*

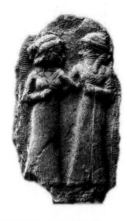

FIGURE 3.6 SACRED UNION OF INANNA AND DUMUZI.

Even thousands of years later, in the Old Testament or Hebrew Bible, we still find traces of erotic hymns. In the Song of Songs (also known as the Song of Solomon), the beautiful Shulamite, the Rose of Sharon, sings to her lover, "Let him kiss me with the kisses of his mouth: for thy love is better than wine. …a bundle of myrrh is my well-beloved unto me; he shall lie all night betwixt my breasts" (Song of Solomon, 1:2, 13, King James translation). And so, the memory of the human body and sexuality as part of the sacred still lingered (Eisler, 1995). Moreover, despite the name "Song of Solomon" given to it by its translators, this section of the Hebrew Bible does not even mention King Solomon—or God.

Archeological excavations also offer important clues to earlier more partnership-oriented societies going back to the early Neolithic (Eisler, 1995). Even though these Neolithic cultures were not ideal, they seem to have had a more egalitarian, peaceful social structure in which women and the feminine were not subordinated to men and the "masculine" (Eisler, 1987, 1995).

Archeological excavations of early Neolithic cultures show few indications of destruction from warfare or of fortifications. Their art does not include images that idealize warfare or rape—again in sharp contrast to the art of later chronically warlike and violent times. While there were some differences in status and in wealth, as the British archeologist James Mellaart (1967) writes, they were not extreme. As the Lithuanian archeologist Marija Gimbutas (1982) and the British archeologist Ian Hodder (2004) write, the evidence also supports the conclusion that women were not subordinate to men.

Hodder (2004) wrote about his excavations of Çatalhöyük in the *Scientific American*. Based on dietary and bone analyses, there are no signs that differences between women and men were translated into differences of status or power. Indeed, as he remarked with some surprise, the evidence suggests a society in which gender is relatively unimportant in assigning social roles.

We want to emphasize this point, as well as the related point that the real alternative to patriarchy is *not* matriarchy (Eisler, 1987). The domination of mothers rather than fathers is simply the other side of a domination coin. The real alternative to both patriarchy and matriarchy is a partnership model of society.

If you move forward in time to the first known high civilization in Europe— the Minoans of Crete—archeological records indicate that a partnership-oriented configuration continued in some places until around 3500 to 4000 years ago. The Minoan civilization was centralized, socially stratified and technologically very advanced, even developing paved roads and indoor plumbing. Yet, as the Greek archeologists Nicolas Platon (1966) and Nano Marinatos (1993) note, there are no signs of destruction by warfare between the various city states on the island of Crete, no hovels contrasting with huge towering fortified palaces for rulers, and, in contrast to the later more domination-oriented Greeks, no slaves.

The Minoans already lived in a world where warfare had become the norm, so we also find weapons and armor. But the Minoan's beautiful art still focused on life and pleasure rather than pain and death.

In Minoan art we find many images of nature, like the so-called dolphin fresco (see Figure 3.7), which could be a modern ecology poster.

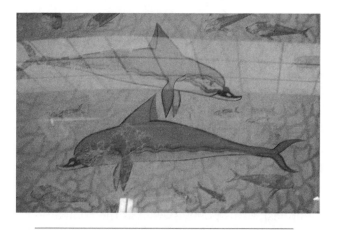

FIGURE 3.7 MINOAN DOLPHIN FRESCO.
(Photo by J. Ollé)

Women are highly sensual, have enormous presence, and are often depicted as priestesses (and men are also sometimes shown as priests; see Figure 3.8). In addition, as Platon (1966) noted, signs of feminine influence as well as of the veneration of a goddess are everywhere.

However, both archeological and mythical records show a shift toward domination systems around 3,500 to 4,000 years ago in this Mediterranean culture. From this time, female figurines appear far less often and signs of destruction through warfare are apparent. Images of battles, conquerors dragging prisoners in chains, and rapes, all absent in the earlier art, became dominant themes as the Minoan culture began to disappear, replaced by Greek influences (Eisler, 1987, 1995).

For example, female deities persisted in the Greek divine pantheon, but they were subordinate to male deities. Democracy was an ideal in ancient Athens, yet it excluded the majority of the population: all women and all slaves. And while the arts were still valued, armed conquest was valued even more (Keuls, 1985)—see Figure 3.9.

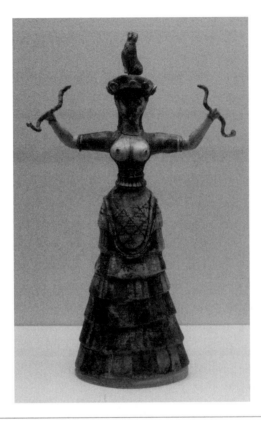

FIGURE 3.8 MINOAN GODDESS OR PRIESTESS.
(Photo by Olaf Tausch)

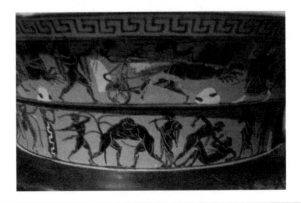

FIGURE 3.9 GREEK VASE IDEALIZING KILLING.
(Photo by Davide Ferro)

The Patterns of History

Viewing cultural evolution from the perspective of the tension between the partnership model and the domination model as two basic possibilities for human societies makes it possible to reevaluate our supposed unilinear evolution from "barbarism" to "civilization." What actually happened suggests a multilinear cultural evolution. That is, in the more fertile areas of the globe, where the earth was a "good mother," more partnership-oriented societies evolved. In the less hospitable areas, the direction was more toward domination (Eisler, 1987, 1995).

This leads to the question of what brought about the shift from a partnership to a domination cultural direction in the early centers of civilization. While many theories exist, there are strong indications that in Europe this shift came about during a period of great disequilibrium marked by invasions from more arid regions. Although some archeologists have claimed that nomadic herders brought civilization to Europe, the archeological record indicates that they actually brought chaos, death, and destruction. As Gimbutas (1982) notes, the Indo-European invaders who took over Europe were people who quite literally worshipped the lethal power of the blade.

What brought these mass migrations into Europe and other fertile areas? One explanation is that extreme climate changes made marginal areas, where herding rather than farming was the main means of subsistence, practically uninhabitable, so hordes of peoples from arid areas gradually took over the more fertile lands and imposed their norms. And once they imposed their domination systems, they radically transformed the direction of cultural evolution (Eisler, 1987, 1995). This appears to have been the case in areas around the Mediterranean, including the Fertile Crescent, which we are taught was the cradle of Western civilization. This was the conclusion of the noted Sumerologist Samuel Noah Kramer who, in *Myths of Enki* (Kramer & Maier, 1989), used Eisler's cultural transformation theory as the explanation for the shift in power to the lugul, or big man, a figure that emerged in Sumerian culture at a time when war between various city-states became the norm.

A similar cultural shift seems to have occurred in other early centers of civilization. For example, after *The Chalice and the Blade* (1987) was published by the Chinese Academy of Social Sciences in Beijing, a group of its Chinese scholars wrote about this in *The Chalice and the Blade in Chinese Culture* (Min, 1995).

Yet even after this massive cultural shift toward domination, the old partnership-based system persisted beneath the surface in the cultural substrate. Moreover, throughout recorded history, there have been partnership resurgences. In the Bible, for instance, there is passage after passage where Jesus preaches partnership values: the stereotypically feminine values of caring, empathy, and peace. In sharp contrast, reflecting a return to domination-based cultural norms, the later Christian church developed as a top-down, rigidly male-dominated, and violent organization (as in its Crusades, Inquisition, and witch burnings).

This tension between movement toward partnership and regressions to domination has punctuated much of recorded history. However, in more recent times the push toward partnership has intensified.

The gradual change from agrarian to industrial modes of production brought increasing technological, economic, and social disequilibrium. This unsettling of old ways of working and living opened the way for renewed movement to the partnership side of the continuum—albeit still against enormous resistance and periodic regressions. Yet if you look at the centuries called *modern history*, you can see this partnership movement gaining strength.

From the perspective of partnership and domination systems as two underlying social possibilities, you can see that all the progressive modern social movements have been challenges to traditions of domination.

- The 17th and 18th century European Enlightenment (also known as the *rights of man movement*) challenged the so-called divinely ordained right of kings to rule.

- The 18th and 19th century feminist movement challenged the so-called divinely ordained right of men to rule women and children in the "castles" of their homes.

- The 19th and 20th century abolitionist, civil rights, and anticolonial movements challenged another supposedly divinely ordained right: that of a "superior" race to rule over "inferior" ones.

- The movements for economic justice and peace and the contemporary movement to end traditions of domination and violence against women and children challenge traditions of top-down economic rule and the use of violence to impose one's will.

- The environmental movement today challenges the conquest and domination of nature.

Table 3.2 draws together some of these domination and partnership examples we've discussed throughout the chapter so you can see the contrasts.

TABLE 3.2 Partnership and Domination Patterns in Prehistory and Ancient History

PARTNERSHIP ILLUSTRATIONS
Stone Age art seems to reflect a society in which the emphasis was on the power to give, nurture, and renew life rather than the power to take life.
The female carvings and sculptures early archeologists called "Venuses" emphasize the life-giving and nurturing powers inherent in women's bodies.
Images of female and male animals as well as vulvas and phalluses are part of their art in ancient cave sanctuaries (Eisler, 1987).
Rather than depicted as prey, the animals in the famous cave paintings are often in pairs of females and males, indicating an understanding that life is the product of the union of female and male.
The Teduray, a 20th century tribal society studied by University of California anthropologist Stuart Schlegel, like our early ancestors, depended largely on gathering and hunting as well as subsistence farming. They valued women and men equally, had elaborate mechanisms for nonviolent conflict resolution, raised children without violence, and respected nature.

"When it came to positive and negative values of human behavior, the same criteria applied to men and women alike" (Schlegel, 1998, p. 111).

"Women and men were clearly different—and the Teduray delighted in the difference. But they were not ranked.... Among forest Teduray neither gender was thought superior to the other in any way. Men and women related with empathy and an ethos of interdependence, with a mutual sharing of life's problems and joys" (Schlegel, 1998, p. 113).

The first followers of Jesus were Jews who questioned authoritarian rule from both their theocratic rulers and their Roman overlords (Akers, 2000; Pagels, 1979; Robinson, 1977).

Many of these sects rejected the ranking of man over woman, and even in the Bible we read of women as apostles and bishops (Acts 2:17, King James translation).

Jesus rebelled against the religious authorities of his time; preached that the meek shall inherit the earth; stopped the stoning of a woman accused of adultery; and, like the Prophet Isaiah before him, urged that we treat others as we would want to be treated by them.

In the Gnostic Gospels, dating to before the Gospels in the Bible, we learn that some early Christians prayed to a Mother and Father and that Mary Magdalene was a major leader in their movement and Jesus's favorite (Pagels, 1979; Robinson, 1977).

DOMINATION ILLUSTRATIONS

The ranking of "superiors" over "inferiors," including the subordination and devaluation of women, is still embedded in many stories we have inherited from earlier more rigid domination times in both the East and West (Eisler, 1987).

Ancient Athens was a slave-holding society where all women were under strict male control. The fabled Athenian democracy applied only to free property-holding men. Women and slaves had little protection under law and custom (Keuls, 1985).

continues

TABLE 3.2 Continued

DOMINATION ILLUSTRATIONS

The famous Greek philosopher Aristotle asserted that women and slaves were meant to be subordinate, or they would not have been born women and slaves. He also wrote, "[T]he relation of male to female is by nature a relation of superior to inferior and ruler to ruled" (Aristotle, trans.1984; Lerner, 1986).

Athenian law and custom ensured women's subordination by denying them education and the right to hold property. (Keuls, 1985)

Ancient Judeo-Christian-Muslim depictions of divine power mirrored a society of top-down rankings: man over man, man over woman, religion over religion, and tribe over tribe (Eisler, 1987).

While there are also passages about peace in the Bible and the Koran, in both, the supreme deity is all-powerful, punitive, and violent, and violence against other groups as well as women is justified as moral (for example, Numbers 31, King James translation; Qur'an 2:191-193). Violence against women if they do not obey their husbands is explicitly justified in the Koran (Qur'an 4:34).

In India, in addition to its famous caste system, women were so devalued that some groups practiced suttee (sati), a custom that decreed that when a man died, his widow was obliged to throw herself into his funeral pyre to be burned alive as a matter of "honor" (Ahmad, 2008).

A recent documentary film features interviews of women about the practice of killing baby girls, which still persists in some world regions such as India and China, and documents the consequent skewed ratio of men to women in these regions (Davis, 2013).

Conclusion

All the modern progressive movements are part of a larger movement toward cultural transformation—this time from domination to partnership (Eisler, 1987, 1995, 2002, 2007). The movement in health care toward interprofessional education and practice, which recognizes the great value of the traditionally female profession of nursing, is an important part of the movement toward the partnership model. Indeed, as we will show in succeeding chapters, nursing is in a unique position to be a key player in this shift.

References

Ahmad, N. (2008). Sati tradition—Widow burning in India: A socio-legal examination. *Web Journal of Current Legal Issues*. Retrieved from http://webjcli.ncl.ac.uk/2009/issue2/ahmad2.html

Akers, K. (2000). *The lost religion of Jesus: Simple living and nonviolence in early Christianity*. New York: Lantern Books.

Bridenthal, R., & Koonz, C. (Eds.). (1977). *Becoming visible: Women in European history*. Boston, MA: Houghton Mifflin.

Conger, J. A., & Kanungo, R. N. (1988). The empowerment process: Integrating theory and practice. *The Academy of Management Review* 13(3), 471-482.

Davis, E. G. (30 July 2013). It's a girl: The three deadliest words in the world. MercatorNet. Retrieved from http://www.mercatornet.com/articles/view/its_a_girl_the_three_deadliest_words_in_the_world#sthash.bbaLR7u2.dpuf

de Waal, F. (2009). *The age of empathy: Nature's lessons for a kinder society*. New York, NY: Harmony Books.

Eisler, R. (1987). *The chalice and the blade: Our history, our future*. San Francisco, CA: HarperCollins.

Eisler, R. (1993). Technology, gender, and history: Toward a nonlinear model of social evolution. In E. Laszlo and I. Masulli, with R. Artigiani & V. Csanyi. (Eds.), *The evolution of cognitive maps: New paradigms for the twenty-first century* (pp. 181-203). Langhorne, PA: Gordon and Breach Science Publishers.

Eisler, R. (1995). *Sacred pleasure: Sex, myth, and the politics of the body*. San Francisco, CA: HarperCollins.

Eisler, R. (1997). Cultural transformation theory: A new paradigm for history. In J. Galtung & S. Inayatullah (Eds.), *Macrohistory and Macrohistorians*. Westport, CN: Praeger Publishers.

Eisler, R. (2000). *Tomorrow's children: A blueprint for partnership education in the 21st century*. Boulder, CO: Westview Press.

Eisler, R. (2002). *The power of partnership: Seven relationships that will change your life*. Novato, CA: New World Library.

Eisler, R. (2003). A multilinear theory of cultural evolution: Genes, culture, and technology. In D. Loye (Ed.), *The great adventure* (pp. 67-98). New York, NY: SUNY Press.

Gilman, C. P. (2007). *Women and economics*. New York, NY: Cosimo.

Gimbutas, M. (1982). *The goddesses and gods of old Europe*. Berkeley, CA: University of California Press.

Hodder, I. (January, 2004). Women and men at Çatalhöyük. *Scientific American, 290*(1), 77-83.

hooks, b. (1984). *Feminist theory: From margin to center*. Boston, MA: South End Press.

Iran Human Rights Documentation Center. (March 8, 2013). *Gender inequality and discrimination: The case of Iranian women*. Retrieved from http://iranhrdc.org/english/publications/legal-commentary/1000000261-gender-inequality-and-discrimination-the-case-of-iranian-women.html#5

Kerber, L. K., & Mathews, J. D. (Eds.). (1982). *Women's America: Refocusing the past*. New York, NY: Oxford University Press.

Keuls, E. (1985). *The reign of the phallus: Sexual politics in ancient Athens*. New York, NY: Harper & Row.

Kramer, S. N., & Maier, J. (1989). *Myths of Enki, the crafty god*. New York, NY: Oxford University Press.

Lerner, G. (1986). *The creation of patriarchy*. New York, NY: Oxford University Press.

Leroi-Gourhan, A. (1971). *Prehistoire de l'Art Occidental*. Paris: Edition D'Art Lucien Mazenod.

Marinatos, N. (1993). *Minoan religion: Ritual, image, and symbol*. Columbia, SC: University of South Carolina Press.

Marshack, A. (1991). *The roots of civilization*. Mount Kisco, NY: Moyer Bell.

Maturana, H., & Varela, F. (1980). *Autopoeisis and cognition: The realization of the living*. Boston, MA: Reidel.

Mellaart, J. (1967). *Çatal Hüyük: A neolithic town in Anatolia*. New York, NY: McGraw-Hill.

Min, J. (Ed.). (1995). *The chalice and the blade in Chinese culture: Gender relations and social models*. Beijing, PRC: China Social Sciences Publishing House.

Niehoff, D. (1999). *The biology of violence: How understanding the brain, behavior, and environment can break the vicious circle of aggression*. New York, NY: Free Press.

Pagels, E, (1979). *The Gnostic gospels*. New York: Random House.

Perry, B. D. (n.d.). Aggression and violence: The neurobiology of experience. Retrieved from http://teacher.scholastic.com/professional/bruceperry/aggression_violence.htm

Platon, N. (1966). *Crete*. Geneva, Switzerland: Nagel Publishers.

Prigogine, I., & Stengers, I. (1984). *Order out of chaos*. New York, NY: Bantam.

Quartz, S. R., & Sejnowski, T. J. (2002). *Liars, lovers, and heroes: What the new brain science reveals about how we become who we are*. New York, NY: Harper Collins.

Robinson, J. (Ed.). (1977). *The Nag Hammadi library in English*. New York, NY: Harper & Row.

Sanday, P. R. (2002). *Women at the center: Life in a modern matriarchy*. Ithaca, New York: Cornell University Press.

Schlegel, S. A. (1998). *Wisdom from a rainforest: The spiritual journey of an anthropologist*. Athens, GA: University of Georgia Press.

Thinkexist.com. (n.d.). *Einstein comment*. Retrieved from http://thinkexist.com/quotation/you-cannot-solve-a-problem-from-the-same/1003327.html

Wolkstein, D., & Kramer, S. N. (1983). *Inanna queen of heaven and earth: Her stories and hymns from Sumer*. New York, NY: Harper & Row.

Chapter 4

The Chalice and the Blade in Nursing

Part I: Early History

"You begin to liquidate a people by taking away its memory. You destroy its books, its culture, its history. And then others write other books for it, give another culture to it, invent another history for it. Then the people slowly begin to forget what it is and what it was. The world at large forgets it still faster."

—*Milan Kundera (1978, p. 218)*

In her 1987 *The Chalice and the Blade*, Eisler examines human history from a broad perspective, allowing her to discern patterns of domination and partnership previously missed by other historians. The history of nursing has similar patterns of domination and partnership, yet these too have been largely overlooked.

In her dissertation, *Reconstructing a New Story of Nursing: Critical Analysis of Nursing Textbooks Using Riane Eisler's Partnership Paradigm,* Potter (2010) analyzes the nursing story found in nursing fundamentals textbooks to deconstruct and expose the limitations of the current story of nursing. As she analyzed the content in the different nursing education texts, Potter sought to answer an important question: Does the current nursing story help perpetuate the subjugation of nurses within a domination model of health care?

Where once greater emphasis was placed on *being* a nurse, modern texts emphasize what nurses *do*. In other words, current texts emphasize nursing actions but ignore nursing presence. This approach fails to socialize nurses to their unique medicine. As you read in Chapter 1, the *BASE of Nursing* (Potter, 2013) demonstrates that the unique medicine of nursing involves *presence*—and even more specifically, using that presence to fully hear the *narratives* of patients, families, and communities. The narratives often hold the key to the most effective care and treatment plans.

When nursing identity is limited to nursing *actions* (scope of practice), the nursing profession risks being externally defined and controlled by others. This is most evident in organizations where hierarchies of domination are in place and nurses are told what to do rather than define their own roles and responsibilities. Losing nursing identity leads to loss of influence and inability to fully partner in interprofessional practice. By contrast, when the meaning of being a nurse is self-determined, external forces cannot diminish the power and influence of nurses.

The real story of nursing demonstrates that nurses have often led the way in improving the quality and experience of care, improving the health of populations, and decreasing the cost of health care. This is both the core of good nursing and the Triple Aim of health care today (Institute for Health Care Improvement [IHI], 2013).

Reexamining Our Professional History

Before you examine the story of nursing, it is important to be aware of some basic definitions. Historian Gerda Lerner (1993) makes a clear distinction between human history and recorded history. *Human history* includes all events, all locations, and all people. It also includes the entire span of time that humans have been a unique species. Human history is both individual and collective, so that both the lives of individuals and the events impacting communities and nations are significant and meaningful. From this more inclusive and holistic perspective, it is easy to see that much of human history has gone unrecorded and has therefore been forgotten.

If human history is intentionally inclusive, recorded history has been purposely exclusive. *Recorded history* represents selective and subjective "remembering." Rather than an objective reporting of historical data, it is the product of a subjective process where selected views, memories, and interpretations are woven into a narrative designed to support a particular ideology. For instance, much of recorded history supports a narrative about the ruling classes—people in power. In fact, you could say that one of the key objectives of recorded history is to rationalize and solidify structures of power or hierarchies of domination. Accordingly, recorded history often includes stories of battles and conquests and justifies the subjugation of one group of people by another.

Recorded histories generally *exclude* the life experiences of those who are disempowered. Therefore, many histories focus on the exploits of men, and few touch upon the traditional world and work of women. The histories fail to record the knowledge and contributions of minorities and those without power (or, at best, give them the barest attention). This is one reason it is difficult to find the recorded history of traditional healers and other ancient roots of nursing.

By contrast, when the meaning of being a nurse is self-determined, external forces cannot diminish their power and influence. The American Association for the History of Nursing's (AAHN) position paper, "Nursing History in the Curriculum: Preparing Nurses for the 21st Century," warns:

> *Nursing does not exist in an unpredictable vacuum. The social pressures that have shaped nursing in the past persist today in new forms. Today's challenges are not easily understood nor addressed in the absence of such insight. This wealth of historical nursing knowledge should not be ignored. (Keeling, 2001, para. 3)*

In short, the story of nursing is more than simply a context for modern nursing. The story of nursing can provide insights and guidance for solving many of today's most pressing health care challenges—hence, the critical importance of reexamining how nursing history is taught.

To better understand the current story of nursing, Potter (2010) used content analysis methodology to analyze the history of nursing content in eight of the most popular nursing fundamental textbooks. Textbooks were selected based on their popularity and their target audience, and they also represent the five major nursing textbook publishers in the United States: Elsevier/Mosby/W. B. Saunders; Wolters Kluwer Health/Lippincott, Williams, and Wilkins; Pearson/Prentice Hall; Thompson/Delmar/Cengage; and F. A. Davis.

In addition, Potter used an earlier nursing textbook, *A Short History of Nursing: From the Earliest Times to the Present Day* by Lavinia Dock and Isabel Stewart (1937) as a control. This approach allowed Potter to compare current nursing ideology with an earlier ideology and to probe the implications for the socialization of novice nurses today.

In her content analysis of Dock and Stewart's (1937) work, Potter found that these early nursing textbook authors seemed to have had a much better sense of the tension between domination and partnership, as indicated by passages such as the following:

> [History] *shows us the long and difficult path by which we have come, and reminds us that continuous progress is by no means an invariable rule in nursing any more than in other human institutions, and that there is always danger of reaction when the nursing spirit grows dim and the forces that make for progress weaken and fail.* (p. 334)

Potter's (2010) content analysis demonstrates that current nursing narratives fail to recognize the powerful impact that domination and partnership have had throughout nursing's history. Commenting on the importance this awareness holds for nurses today, she wrote:

> *It is important for nurses to know that progress is an active process requiring nursing leadership and vision to make certain that future*

*healthcare models are not only effective but also sustainable.
Nurses also need to be aware that opposing forces are always
present and need to be creatively addressed. The tension between
domination and partnership values has been a major thread of the
history of nursing and most likely will continue to be part of the
nursing context for years to come. (p. 111)*

Potter (2010) concluded that current textbooks perhaps unintentionally
continue to reinforce a domination narrative, not only because they exclude
the full history of nursing, but also because of the words, exemplars, and
photographs that they include. For example, autonomous nursing roles such as
nurse-led models of care and nursing midwifery were excluded from most of
the texts, reinforcing the message that nursing practice is always dependent on
hospitals and physicians.

Of particular relevance to the future of nursing, Potter (2010) found the
textbooks failed to adequately prepare nurses for interprofessional practice.
The texts not only neglected to provide examples of historical partnerships
between nurses and other providers, they also only minimally touched upon the
collaborative skills currently required in health care.

Once gaps in the current story of nursing became evident, Potter (2010) used
Eisler's (1987) cultural transformation theory and autobiographical writings of
historic nurse exemplars to create an alternative narrative, one that empowers
nurses to be full partners in health care. The story that follows is based on
Potter's 2010 dissertation *Reconstructing a New Story of Nursing: Critical
Analysis of Nursing Textbooks Using Riane Eisler's Partnership Paradigm.*

The Chalice and the Blade in Nursing: Early History

"The universe is made of stories, not of atoms."
—*Muriel Rukeyser (1968, p. 111)*

A great teaching comes from the ancient indigenous people of West Africa: "It is
not wrong to go back for that which you have forgotten" (The Spirituals Project,

2004, para. 5). Half a world away, the indigenous Anishnabe of North America received a similar message in the Seven Fires Prophecy: "At the time of the Seventh Fire, a new people will emerge. They will retrace the footsteps of their ancestors to find those things that have been lost along the way" (Dostou, 2000, para. 15).

Many indigenous people recognize the wisdom of their ancestors and the important lessons they can learn from their past. This value is not about returning to live the way we did in the past: It reflects the understanding that knowledge from the past may still be beneficial today. As noted earlier in this chapter, the American Association for the History of Nursing concurs, stating that nursing history can expand our thinking, offer solutions for current health care challenges, and provide nurses with a strong sense of professional identity (Keeling, 2001).

Nurses need to ask, "Is there something we have forgotten? Can stories of our nursing ancestors both inspire and inform our practice today?"

Throughout history, forces have attempted to control and contain people who provided care for those in need; however, many historic nurses refused to be defined by others. These ordinary women and men challenged oppressive forces to accomplish extraordinary things. Their words and stories remind us of something we may have forgotten—*nurses are full partners in healing.*

The following story of nursing illuminates historic patterns of subjugation and partnership through the words and stories of historic nurses. May the stories inform us, enlighten us, and inspire us to collaborate for better care.

In the Beginning

Most stories of modern nursing begin with either Florence Nightingale or the ancient Greeks and Romans. But if you start at either of these points, you miss 99% of the story (Shostak, 1981). The real story of nursing begins with our most ancient human ancestors. Written accounts don't exist of that time, but you can make inferences from myths, archeological records, and some contemporary gathering-hunting cultures.

People who speak the ancient click-based Khoisan language are known by many names: !Kung, San, Ju/'hoansi, and Bushmen. They are the surviving remnants of humanity's earliest genetic line (Rincon, 2008; Wells, 2002). Indeed, modern San Bushmen may be seen as keepers of the oldest healing traditions on earth (Keeney, 1999). Stories from traditional !Kung healers offer insights about humanity's first healing paradigm, and these values and beliefs may also represent the earliest roots of nursing.

Dr. Bradford Keeney (1999, 2003) extensively interviewed the !Kung traditional healers (N/om-Kxaosi) and recorded descriptions of the healer's role and !Kung cosmology. Keeney's interviews provide important insights, since most cultures rooted in oral tradition use stories to efficiently and accurately pass knowledge from generation to generation (Vansina, 1985). According to Keeney (1999), the !Kung do not use healing practices based on a written or oral tradition. Instead they are directly connected to *n/om*, which is the life force or spirit. The N/om-Kxaosi are in relationship with *n/om* and this allows them to heal the whole person. This healing power of *n/om* is a lost thread in evidence-based practice curriculum, yet personal stories indicate it is still a driving force for many holistic nurses.

NOTE

According to the American Holistic Nurses Association (AHNA), "The practice of holistic nursing requires nurses to integrate self-care, self-responsibility, spirituality, and reflection in their lives. This may lead the nurse to greater awareness of the interconnectedness with self, others, nature, and spirit. This awareness may further enhance the nurses understanding of all individuals and their relationships to the human and global community, and permits nurses to use this awareness to facilitate the healing process" (2013).

Content analysis of Keeney's interviews with the N/om-Kxaosi reveal recurring themes in the !Kung healing paradigm, including the following:

- There is a connection between our emotional state and our state of physical health.

- Having an open heart and intense feelings of compassion are important qualities for a healer.

- Different ways of knowing are acknowledged and respected.

- Healing modalities include song, dance, touch, shaking, and stories.

- Healing occurs at the community level as well as the individual level, and frequently there is no distinction between the two.

- Healing involves transformation and change. (Keeney, 1999, 2003)

Our earliest human ancestors thus seem to have embraced a holistic understanding of health and healing. The earliest people, as well as a number of indigenous people today, did not see a separation between cure and care, mind and body, spirit and material, science and art. All things past and present are part of the web of life that surrounds us and supports us. (See Figure 4.1.)

The *web of life* is not a quaint metaphor for the !Kung: The N/om-Kxaosi actually see, feel, and travel along the lines that interconnect all things (Keeney, 2003). The Bushmen healers also use these connecting lines to send thoughts to others. They use the medicine of shaking love to strengthen the web of connections so it will support future generations. A great deal of information about the health and wellness of individuals and the community comes from the healers' ability to sense the quality of the connecting lines (Keeney, 2003).

Another source of knowledge comes through acute observation. The N/om-Kxaosi reported:

We watch animals, especially the gemsbok [antelope], to see what medicines they use. We study their stomach contents and watch what plants they eat. Then we try them ourselves. This is how we learned about some of the medicines of the world. The gemsbok and other wild animals have taught us many things about healing one another. They show us what medicines to use. (Keeney, 1999, p. 31)

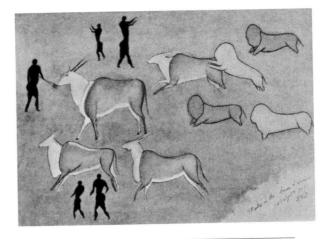

FIGURE 4.1 SOUTH AFRICAN ROCK ART.
(Photographer: George William Stow [1822-1882])

Bushmen healers expertly blend the art and science of healing. They also maintain the threads of interconnection among community members, the environment, and the spirits. The role of the N/om-Kxao, or traditional healer, is not fragmented into treatment provider and care provider (Keeney, 1999). It appears caring is the treatment and the treatment is caring; both are performed by the same healer. !Kung men and women have different songs and dances and report different experiences related to healing, but the role of healer is not based on gender (Keeney, 1999). Anthropology professor Barbara Tedlock reaches a similar conclusion in *The Woman in the Shaman's Body* (2005). She presents archeological evidence from around the globe that indicates both men and women were respected traditional healers during the Paleolithic era or prehistory. Artificial splitting and ranking of the healer's role along gender lines occurred much later.

!Kung would also not understand our modern separation of public health and individual health. For them, the individual's health is a manifestation of the health of the community, and the health of the community is directly connected to the health of each individual.

Ju/'hoan healing involves health and growth on physical, psychological, social, and spiritual levels; it affects the individual, the group, the surrounding environment, and the cosmos. Healing is an integrating and enhancing force, touching far more levels and forces than simply caring for an individual's illness. (Katz, Biesele, & St. Denis, 1997, p. 1)

We need to recover this lost thread of *whole systems healing* (Kreitzer, 2012) if the current health care system is to truly be reformed.

One final lesson from the !Kung is the importance of partnership and collaboration. The !Kung are not perfect, their societies are not ideal, and their lives are certainly not free from challenges. But their gathering-hunting lifestyle based on shared resources, egalitarian relationships, and mutual goals offers an example of a culture that is more oriented toward partnership.

Katz et al. (1997) reported that the Ju/'hoansi do not own resources nor do they defend territories; in their culture, sharing with others is a fundamental value taught to children. For example, "children learn that part of whatever is put into one of their hands must immediately go out the other hand to someone else. Equalizing and leveling are two main themes in the Ju/'hoan society" (p. 51). Shostak (1981) reports, "Most childhood games involve little or no competition.... But !Kung adults also actively avoid competition and the ranking of individuals into hierarchies" (p. 98). !Kung relationships are thus primarily based on collaboration. The community avoids creating a fear of scarcity; therefore, members trust their needs will be met. Adopting this value could impact modern society's epidemic levels of stress and stress-related diseases.

However, we must be careful not to overly romanticize belief systems and healing traditions from indigenous cultures. In fact, some early gatherer-hunter cultures and some modern indigenous cultures are organized according to principles of domination. Traditional healing knowledge is not always beneficial and can actually be harmful. Furthermore, fear and ignorance can thwart life-sustaining public health initiatives. To illustrate, recently, in Pakistan a United Nations-backed polio-eradication campaign had to be suspended when militant gunmen shot and killed a female worker, alleging that the health care workers were U.S. spies and that the vaccines would cause sterility (Khan & Toosi, 2013).

Rather, the point is that our current culture has dismissed as "old" beliefs, values, and knowledge that may be beneficial today. The following discussion explains how these "missing" values are often found in the partnership paradigm. The degree to which a culture or society aligns with the principles of partnership determines its value for the nursing narrative.

Civilization and the Rise of Domination Systems

In Chapter 3 of this book Eisler describes patterns of partnership and domination in early prehistory and history. Potter (2010) used Eisler's model and uncovered similar patterns related to early healers. These patterns are discussed here.

Scholars say that many factors prompted cultures moving away from gatherer-hunter lifestyles to more permanent settlements organized around agriculture. Despite that change, partnership values persisted. Consider prehistoric Anatolian (Turkish) city of Çatal Hüyük (6250–5720 BCE). It is estimated that between 6,000 and 8,000 people lived in this important town, one of the first large, permanent settlements organized around agriculture. There are no signs of destruction from warfare. Neither houses nor grave goods indicate large distinctions in status or wealth. According to archeologist Ian Hodder (2004), dietary and bone analyses show no signs that differences between women and men were translated into differences of status or power. In summary, there is no evidence of hierarchies of domination, male dominance, or war (Eisler, 1987; Lerner, 1986; Mellaart, 1967). You can find this kind of cultural organization in other Neolithic sites, including a large number of excavations in the area archeologist Marija Gimbutas (1974, 1991) called "Old Europe." These sites revealed the existence of similar models of ancient civilization. For instance, from 7000–3500 BCE in the area of the Balkan Peninsula, complex egalitarian horticulturalist communities were structured more like the gatherer-hunters. Both genders performed tasks essential for group survival (Eisler, 1987; Gimbutas, 1974, 1991). In such societies the genders were considered complementary— roles being different but equal (Lerner, 1986).

Eisler (1987) wrote that in Old Europe where the Great Goddess was worshipped, "the primary purpose of art, and of life, was not to conquer, pillage, and loot but to cultivate the earth and provide the material and spiritual wherewithal for a satisfying life" (p. 20). Religious symbols found at archeological excavation sites were related to nature's cycles of birth, death, and regeneration rather than war. Related to healing, grave contents from ancient sites in Denmark indicated that women might have been important shamanic healers. Achterberg (1990) wrote, "Women were omnipotent in myth, cherished for their connection to nature, regarded as healers, and believed to hold power in the invisible realm" (p. 28).

Things changed dramatically, however, when nomadic people—whom Gimbutas calls the Kurgans because they brought with them a new method of burial called *kurgan*—overran the indigenous European communities (Eisler, 1987, 1995; Gimbutas, 1974, 1991). The Kurgans were Indo-European tribes from the Russian Steppes who swept into Europe in three different waves (see Figure 4.2).

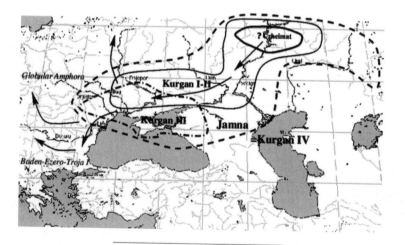

FIGURE 4.2 KURGAN MAP.
(Source: Created by Dbachmann)

Now gods of thunder and war replaced the Great Goddess of nature (Eisler, 1987; Gimbutas, 1974, 1991; Keller, 1996). Gimbutas summarized the radical difference between the Old European and Kurgan systems of social organization:

The Old European and Kurgan cultures were the antithesis of one another. The Old Europeans were sedentary horticulturalists prone to live in well-planned townships. The absence of fortifications and weapons attests the peaceful coexistence of this egalitarian society that was probably matrilineal and matrilocal. The Kurgan system was composed of patrilineal, socially stratified, herding units, which lived in small villages or seasonal settlements while grazing their animals over vast areas. One economy based on farming, the other on stock breeding and grazing, produced two contrasting ideologies. The Old European belief system focused on the agricultural cycle of birth, death, and regeneration, embodied in the female principle, the Mother Creatrix. The Kurgan ideology, as known from comparative Indo-European mythology, exalted virile, heroic warrior gods of the shining and thunderous sky. Weapons are nonexistent in Old European imagery; whereas the dagger and battle-axe are dominant symbols of the Kurgans, who like all historically known Indo-Europeans glorified the power of the sharp blade. (Gimbutas as quoted in Eisler, 1987, p. 48)

The overthrow of what Eisler calls "the culture of the chalice" by "the culture of the blade" (1987) had powerful implications for healers that can still be felt today. Domination brought ranking of man over man, man over woman, race over race, religion over religion, and man over nature. The holistic thinking of partnership disappeared and was replaced with dualistic thinking (Achterberg, 1990).

For example, in Mesopotamia the role of the healer was split into two distinct professions, the *ashipu* and the *asu* (Price, 2001). The *ashipu* in older texts was known as a witch doctor or sorcerer—the healer responsible for diagnosing the illness and determining which god or demon was responsible. The *ashipu*'s treatments included spells and charms to protect the patient and restore health. The *asu*, on the other hand, specialized in herbal remedies and was often referred to as a physician. The *asu*'s treatments included bandaging, plasters, and care of wounds (Price, 2001). Initially the *ashipu* and *asu* were equally valued in Sumer (Achterberg, 1990), but that later changed under the domination system. The role of the healer, which was holistic for much of human history, was now split, with different roles assigned and ranked according to gender.

Eisler (1987) holds that in the shift to a domination system, social roles associated with power became exclusively male. Therefore, diagnosing and prescribing treatments were assigned to males because these skills were associated with education and power; caring was not associated with either power or prestige, so it was assigned to females.

This shift in the healing professions was part of a larger shift in how people saw the world. For much of human history, people believed that the Great Goddess ruled the heavens and earth. Lerner (1986) wrote, "There was unity among earth and the stars, humans and nature, birth and death, all of which were embodied in the Great Goddess" (p. 148). Now the original myths about creation and the realm of spirit changed: In the new myth, a male god presided over a hierarchy that ranked certain males over all other humans.

Teachings of the Great Faiths

In the previous chapter of this book, Eisler used both historical and cross-cultural data to demonstrate a historical tension between two underlying models of social organization. The domination model, based on rigid hierarchies of control, is ultimately maintained through violence or the threat of violence. The partnership model, based on respect and mutuality, seeks to connect and empower each member of the community.

Stepping back, you begin to see that the history of healing also includes patterns of domination and partnership. Even though Goddess and nature myths were erased or rewritten with the arrival of cultures of domination, many of the early spiritual teachings continued to challenge systems of domination. The Hindu Vedas (1500–500 BCE), for example, contain passages such as, "The physician, the drugs, the attendant, and the patient constitute the four basic factors of treatment … they lead to the earliest cure of diseases" (Ghai & Ghai, 1997, p. 131). In these ancient Indian scripts there was no hierarchy of cure over care; the physician, the attendant (or nurse), and the patient were equally important for healing.

You can find another example in Buddhism, the texts of which originate as early as 1000 BCE. In this spiritual tradition, the *bodhisattva*, or enlightened being, made 12 vows that came to be known as the "Medicine Buddha Sutra" (Thanh & Leigh, 2001). The Tenth Vow, which is significant for this discussion, states:

> *I vow that in a future life when I have attained Supreme Enlightenment, those sentient beings who are shackled, beaten, imprisoned, condemned to death or otherwise subjected to countless miseries and humiliations by royal decree—and who are suffering in body and mind from this oppression—need only hear my name to be freed from these afflictions. (p. 22)*

In this sutra, the Buddha challenges subjugation and vows to intervene to free the oppressed.

As Eisler points out, Christianity and Judaism also contain partnership teachings. Achterberg (1990) reported, "Jesus himself challenged the religious and social institutions of his day with a frontal assault on patriarchy, shocking his contemporaries with his open consort with and esteem for women" (p. 38). (See Figure 4.3.) In the Bible, early followers of Jesus were told by Apostle Paul, "There is neither Jew nor Greek, slave nor free, male nor female, for you are all one in Christ Jesus" (Galatians 3:28, New International Version). The earliest followers of the Christian belief system also based their communities on partnership rather than domination.

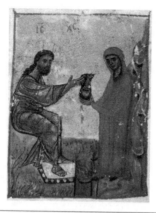

FIGURE 4.3 JESUS AND THE WOMAN AT THE WELL.
(Source: Center of Manuscripts [Tbilisi, Georgia])

Similarly, in Islam the Holy Qur'an (Koran) teaches followers to recognize "the connections between knowledge, health, holism, the environment, and the 'Oneness of Allah,' the unity of God in all spheres of life, death, and the hereafter" (Rassool, 2000, p. 1476).

The great faith systems attempted to offer an alternative to fragmentation and systems of domination; unfortunately, as Eisler (1987) documents, religious scriptures also reflect the domination culture of their time. At the core of these great faiths, however, lie partnership values such as caring, empathy, and nonviolence. Systems of domination stereotype these values as feminine, hence, having no real power. Yet early nurses knew differently.

The Code of Hospitality and the Deaconess Movement

The partnership teachings of the great faiths impacted nursing in significant ways. Common values among the great faiths include compassion, caring for others, and the belief that physical health is strongly connected to spiritual health. These teachings provided inspiration for many early forms of nursing service.

For instance, hospitality was an important value in many early partnership-based cultures from gatherer-hunters to ancient agrarian communities. Lerner (1986) writes, "Among desert nomads, a lone individual cannot survive; thus hospitality to a stranger was a basic and sacred rule" (p. 163). The values of compassion and hospitality may have prompted establishment of hospitals where travelers and people without families could receive care in times of need.

Achterberg (1990) reported that in 394 CE (Common Era) Fabiola, a wealthy Roman patrician and convert to Christianity, established one of the earliest public hospitals in the West. Spiritual faith inspired women who established early hospitals in Arabia, too. Al-Hashmi (as cited in Jan, 1996) wrote, "With the permission of Prophet Mohammed, Rufaida raised her tent inside the mosque to provide care as well as health education" (p. 267). Rufaida Al-Asamiya was also noted for establishing the first school of nursing for women (Jan, 1996), more than 1,200 years before Florence Nightingale.

Another application of the spiritual call to be a nurse was seen in the deaconess movement. The New Testament says that early Christian communities shared property and participated in communal meals. The deacons were followers specifically called to provide care for the community's widows, orphans, poor, and afflicted. Male and female deacons were respected equally for their caring service (Golder, 1903). The deaconess movement provided services to the poor and sick up until the 13th century, when the pendulum again swung sharply toward domination.

Even though individual Christians may have lived closer to principles of partnership, the Orthodox Church not only formed an alliance with the Roman Emperor but also moved toward the domination side of the partnership/ domination continuum. Three hundred years after the death of Jesus, women were ousted from their earlier leadership positions and decreed subordinate to men; "heretics" (including competing Jewish and Christian sects) were persecuted and killed; and the Church became rigidly male-dominated, violent, and authoritarian—the kind of domination system Jesus had preached against (Eisler, 1987).

The Inquisition

The Inquisition was one of the most tragic chapters in the history of nursing, and it is critical that nurses today grasp what happened to female healers during the European Middle Ages. Eisler (1987) writes:

> *The burning and persecution of heretics, those who did not perceive reality in the prescribed way were killed or converted… through intermittent social shows of force such as public inquisitions and executions, behaviors, attitudes, and perceptions that did not conform to dominator norms were systematically discouraged. This fear conditioning became part of all aspects of daily life, permeating child rearing, laws, and schools. (p. 83)*

The documented reticence of modern nurses to speak publicly about health care issues (Buresh & Gordon, 2000) and their frequent refusal to challenge the current health care system may be directly related to this fear conditioning.

During the Middle Ages, the wealthy could afford to hire physicians, while the poor and outcast sought remedies from the village "wise woman" (Achterberg, 1990). These wise women "functioned as herbalists and empiricists, sustaining the healing lore through oral tradition and apprenticeship. They did what women always do—sit at the bedside and work with whatever ingredients and rituals are available to ease pain and suffering" (Achterberg, 1990, p. 42).

In *Witches, Midwives, and Nurses: A History of Women Healers,* Ehrenreich and English (1973) wrote of the intentional suppression of female healers during the Middle Ages:

> *The suppression of women health workers and the rise to dominance of male professionals was not a 'natural' process, resulting automatically from changes in medical science, nor was it the result of women's failure to take on healing work. It was an active takeover by male professionals…. The stakes of the struggle were high: Political and economic monopolization of medicine meant control over its institutional organizations, its theory and practice, its profits and prestige. (p. 4)*

The domination paradigm was most evident during the witch trials where thousands of traditional healers, mostly herbalists and midwives, were murdered (Ehrenreich & English, 1973). Abram (1996) stated that the Inquisition (Figure 4.4) reflects "the attempted, and near successful, extermination of the last orally preserved traditions of Europe" (p. 199).

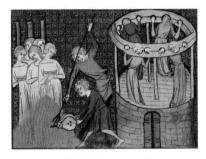

FIGURE 4.4 THE INQUISITION AND WITCH BURNING.

According to Ehrenreich and English (1973), the two forces responsible for these years of massacres were the ruling Church authorities and the emerging European medical profession. The *Malleus Maleficarum*, or Hammer of Witches, published in 1486 by Reverends Kramer and Sprenger, was the authoritative text for conducting witch trials. This text stated that one of the primary ways to determine whether or not an illness was caused by a witch, rather than a natural cause, was to consult a physician (Achterberg, 1990; Ehrenreich & English, 1973).

The "wise women" or folk healers were not only accused of causing harm, but sometimes their fault lay in their success. Achterberg (1990) wrote, "They were accused of the 'crimes' of aiding the sick, birthing babies, and caring for the dying. In areas where the emergent male professionals had their greatest strength, many of these women were accused of witchcraft" (p. 89). These women healers were excluded from formal education; therefore, their healing knowledge was acquired through oral tradition, apprenticeship, and direct experience (similar to many indigenous medical people).

The chief threat for the Church and medical profession was that these healers practiced autonomously. Consider the case of Jacoba Felicie:

> *Brought to trial in 1322 by the faculty of Medicine at the University of Paris…. The primary accusations brought against her were that she would cure her patient of internal illness and wounds or of external abscesses. She would visit the sick assiduously and continue to examine the urine in the manner of physicians, feel the pulse, and touch the body and limbs. (Ehrenreich & English, 1973, p. 18)*

This case indicates that some of these women healers were burned alive for caring for the sick using the same skills practiced by nurses today.

Conclusion

The reason nurses are currently able to provide care for the ill and poor without threat of harm can be credited to nurses who later courageously challenged the domination paradigm. It is with the inspiring stories of some of these nurses that we will in the next chapter continue our reexamination of the important and all too often ignored history of nursing.

References

Abram, D. (1996). *The spell of the sensuous: Perception and Language in a More-Than-Human World.* New York, NY: Vintage Books.

Achterberg, J. (1990). *Woman as healer.* Boston, MA: Shambhala.

American Holistic Nurses Association (AHNA). (2013). What is holistic nursing? Retrieved from http://www.ahna.org/AboutUs/WhatisHolisticNursing/tabid/1165/Default.aspx

Buresh, B., & Gordon, S. (2000). *From silence to voice: What nurses know and must communicate to the public.* Ithaca, NY: Cornell University Press.

Dock, L. L., & Stewart, I. M. (1937). *A short history of nursing: From the earliest times to the present day,* Third Edition. New York, NY: G.P. Putnam's Sons.

Dostou, T. (2000). Seven fires prophecy of the Anishnabe people and the process of reconciliation. Retrieved from http://www.oneprayer.org/Seven_Fires_Prophecy.html

Ehrenreich, B., & English, D. (1973). *Witches, midwives and nurses: A history of women healers.* New York, NY: Feminist Press at the City University of New York.

Eisler, R. (1987). *The chalice and the blade: Our history, our future.* San Francisco, CA: Harper & Row.

Eisler, R. (1995). *Sacred pleasure: Sex, myth, and the politics of the body.* San Francisco, CA: HarperCollins.

Ghai, S., & Ghai, C. M. (1997). The ancient origin of nursing in India. *Nursing Journal of India, 88*(6), 131–132.

Gimbutas, M. (1974). *The gods and goddesses of old Europe: 7000–3500 BCE.* London, UK: Thames & Hudson.

Gimbutas, M. (1991). *The civilization of the goddess: The world of old Europe.* San Francisco, CA: HarperSanFrancisco.

Golder, C. (1903). *History of the deaconess movement in the Christian church.* Cincinnati, OH: Jennings & Pye.

Hodder, I. (2004). Women and men at Çatalhöyük. *Scientific American, 290*(1), 77-83.

Institute for Health Care Improvement (IHI). (2013). IHI Triple Aim Initiative. Retrieved from http://www.ihi.org/offerings/initiatives/tripleaim/Pages/default.aspx

Jan, R. (1996). Rufaida Al-Asalmiya: The first Muslim nurse. *Journal of Nursing Scholarship, 28*(3), 267-268.

Katz, R., Biesele, M., & St. Denis, V. (1997). *Healing makes our hearts happy: Spirituality and cultural transformation among the Kalahari Ju/'hoansi.* Rochester VT: Inner Traditions.

Keeling, A. (2001). Nursing history in the curriculum: Preparing nurses for the 21st century. Retrieved from http://www.aahn.org/position.html

Keeney, B. (1999). *Kalahari bushmen healers.* Philadelphia, PA: Ringing Rocks Press.

Keeney, B. (2003). *Ropes to God: Experiencing the bushman spiritual universe.* Philadelphia, PA: Ringing Rocks Press.

Keller, M. L. (1996). Gimbutas's theory of early European origins and the contemporary transformation of western civilization. *Journal of Feminist Studies in Religion, 12*(2), 73-90.

Khan, R., & Toosi, N. (2013, May 29). Pakistan suspends vaccine effort. *StarTribune,* p. A4.

Kreitzer, M. J. (2012). Whole systems healing. Retrieved from http://www.csh.umn.edu/wsh/

Kundera, M. (1978). *The book of laughter and forgetting.* New York, NY: HarperPerennial.

Lerner, G. (1986). *The creation of patriarchy.* New York, NY: Oxford University Press.

Lerner, G. (1993). *The creation of feminist consciousness: From the Middle Ages to eighteen-seventy.* New York, NY: Oxford University Press.

Mellaart, J. (1967). *Çatal Hüyük: A Neolithic Town in Anatolia.* New York, NY: McGraw-Hill.

Potter, T. M. (2010). Reconstructing a new story of nursing: Critical analysis of nursing textbooks using Riane Eisler's partnership paradigm. *Dissertation Abstracts International,* 72(05), 3447086.

Potter, T. M. (2013). *The BASE of nursing.* Unpublished manuscript, School of Nursing, University of Minnesota, United States of America.

Price, M. (2001, October). History of ancient medicine in Mesopotamia and Iran. Retrieved from http://www.iranchamber.com/history/articles/ancient_medicine_mesopotamia_iran.php

Rassool, G. H. (2000). The crescent and Islam: Healing, nursing, and the spiritual dimension. Some considerations towards an understanding of the Islamic perspectives on caring. *Journal of Advanced Nursing, 32*(6), 1476-1484.

Rincon, P. (2008). Human line 'nearly split in two.' *BBC News.* Retrieved from http://news.bbc.co.uk/2/hi/science/nature/7358868.stm

Rukeyser, M. (1968). *The speed of darkness.* New York, NY: Random House.

Shostak, M. (1981). *Nisa: The life and words of a !Kung woman.* Cambridge, MA: Harvard University Press.

Tedlock, B. (2005). *The woman in the shaman's body: Reclaiming the feminine in religion and medicine.* New York, NY: Bantam.

Thanh, M., & Leigh, P. D. (2001). Sutra of the medicine Buddha. North Hills, CA: International Buddhist Monastic Institute. Retrieved from http://www.buddhanet.net/pdf_file/medbudsutra.pdf

The Spirituals Project. (2004). African traditions, proverbs, and Sankofa. Retrieved from University of Denver's Center for Teaching and Learning, Spirituals Project website: http://ctl.du.edu/spirituals/Literature/sankofa.cfm

Vansina, J. (1985). *Oral tradition as history.* Madison, WI: University of Wisconsin Press.

Wells, S. (2002). *The journey of man: A genetic odyssey.* Princeton, NJ: Princeton University Press.

Chapter 5

The Chalice and the Blade in Nursing

Part II: Modern Exemplars of Partnership-Based Nursing

"The stories people tell have a way of taking care of them. If stories come to you, care for them. And learn to give them away where they are needed. Sometimes a person needs a story more than food to stay alive. That is why we put these stories in each other's memories. This is how people care for themselves."

–Barry Lopez (1990)

The first part of "The Chalice and the Blade in Nursing" (see Chapter 4) identifies patterns of domination and partnership that have shaped and impacted nursing throughout history. This chapter continues the story of nursing with narratives about nurses who chose to be *partners in healing*.

What follows is again based on Potter's (2010) dissertation, *Reconstructing a New Story of Nursing: Critical Analysis of Nursing Textbooks Using Riane Eisler's Partnership Paradigm*.

The Chalice and the Blade in Nursing: Partners in Healing

The following selections from a number of autobiographies indicate that even in the midst of systems of domination, the partnership paradigm was a guiding influence in the lives and work of many nursing pioneers. The autobiographies also provide evidence that these early nurses considered presence and listening to narratives to be important parts of their care. Even though the work that nurses do has changed over time, the medicine of nursing is timeless.

Mary Seacole (1805-1881)

"See here is Mary Seacole, who did as much in the Crimea as another magic-lamping Lady, but being dark could scarce be seen for the flame of Florence's candle."

–Salman Rushdie (1988, p. 301)

Most nurses are familiar with Florence Nightingale's work in the Crimea, yet few people recognize the name Mary Seacole. Seacole triumphed over prejudice and subjugation to courageously provide care and medicine to soldiers on the battlefield.

Seacole was a Creole "doctress" from Jamaica. She learned herbal and traditional African folk medicine from her mother, who managed a boarding house for disabled British soldiers. Traditional healers did not split care and cure; therefore, Seacole combined both in her healing ministry. She was just as apt to dress a wound and care for a feverish patient as she was to reach into her medicine bag for an effective herbal treatment (Seacole, 1857/2005). Early in Seacole's career, she gained recognition for the care she provided for British soldiers suffering from cholera and dysentery in Panama. When she read newspaper reports of the terrible conditions and high mortality rate of British soldiers fighting in the Crimean War, she immediately left for London. She knew her healing skills and herbal knowledge would help save lives in the Crimea (Seacole, 1857/2005).

In her autobiography, *Wonderful Adventures of Mrs. Seacole in Many Lands* (1857/2005), Seacole described a transformative encounter with the domination system:

> *Feeling that I was one of the very women most wanted, experienced, fond of work, I jumped at once to the conclusion that they would gladly enroll me in their number…. I had an interview with one of Miss Nightingale's companions …. I read in her face the fact, that had there been a vacancy, I should not have been chosen to fill it…. I was so conscious of the unselfishness of the motives which induced me to leave England—so certain of the service I could render among the sick soldiery, and yet I found it so difficult to convince others of these facts…. Did these ladies shrink from accepting aid because my blood flowed beneath a somewhat duskier skin than theirs? Tears streamed down my foolish cheeks, as I stood in the fast thinning streets; tears of grief that any should doubt my motives—that heaven should deny my opportunity that I sought. Then I stood still, and looking upward through and through the dark clouds that shadowed London, prayed aloud for help…. Let what might happen, to the Crimea I would go…. I would have willingly given my services as a nurse; but as they declined them, should I not go and open a hotel for invalids in the Crimea in my own way? (pp. 73-74)*

The hierarchy of the domination system excluded Seacole despite her obvious qualifications. But fortunately, she trusted her own sense of calling. When the traditional route of service was barred, she creatively forged another path.

Seacole borrowed money and traveled alone to the Crimea. When she arrived, she discovered that the British hospital, managed by Nightingale, was in Scutari on the opposite shore of the Black Sea, far from the Crimean battlefront.

Therefore, Seacole decided to move to the Crimean peninsula near Sevastopol, a few miles from the front. There she sold merchandise and provisions to the military and offered a place for respite for the officers (Seacole, 1857/2005).

In her autobiography, Seacole reported that a "little bird" regularly informed her about the location of the next day's battle. She would load up her wagon with medicines and bandages, travel to the battle, and—often under fire—care for the injured and dying. She did not honor one uniform over another, caring for Russian infantrymen as regularly as fallen British officers (Seacole, 2005).

The greatest testimony to a nurse's skill comes not from fellow professionals, but from the patients the nurse serves. Here is a patient's testimony regarding Seacole:

> *I certify that I was labouring under a severe attack of diarrhoea last August, and that I was restored to health through the instrumentality and kindness of Mrs. Seacole. I also certify that my fingers were severely jammed whilst at work on Frenchman's Hill, and Mrs. Seacole cured me after three doctors had fruitlessly attempted to cure them. And I cannot leave the Crimea without testifying to the kindness and skill of Mrs. Seacole and may God reward her for it.*
>
> *–James Wallen, 5th Division, Army Work Corps (p. 115)*

Seacole's autobiography concludes with numerous letters reflecting similar gratitude. Obviously, these soldiers appreciated that Seacole trusted her sense of calling.

These words summarize Seacole's philosophy of care: "I love to be of service … And wherever the need arises—on whatever distant shore—I ask no greater or higher privilege than to minister to it" (Seacole, 1857/2005, p. 31).

Florence Nightingale (1820-1910)

Florence Nightingale is recognized for her work in the Crimea, where she was able to dramatically decrease the death rate of British soldiers by efficiently managing the hospital environment. In many ways, Nightingale was an expert hospital administrator. In addition, she was well trained in statistics and used this skill to demonstrate the effectiveness of her interventions (Bostridge, 2008).

While Nightingale believed that nursing was different from—but equal to—medicine, the medical establishment was very pleased with her model of nursing care. The Nightingale model did not appear to threaten their territory. Despite Nightingale's work, public and medical establishments were still unable to break free of the domination paradigm's rigid hierarchies. In her classic work *Notes on Nursing: What It Is and What It Is Not* (1860/1969), Nightingale acknowledged this: "So deep-rooted and universal is the conviction that to give medicine is to be doing something, rather everything; to give air, warmth, cleanliness, etc., is to do nothing" (p. 9). Nightingale realized, however, that attention to the environment, including air, cleanliness, light, warmth, food, and levels of noise, is essential to healing (Nightingale, 1860/1969).

Not only was Nightingale (1860/1969) aware of the inequality between the two branches of healing, she was also acutely aware of the subjugation of nurses by physicians. She wrote:

I have often seen good nurses distressed, because they could not impress the doctor with the real danger of their patient.... The distress is very legitimate, but it generally arises from the nurse not having the power of laying clearly and shortly before the doctor the facts from which she derives her opinion, or from the doctor being hasty and inexperienced, and not capable of eliciting them. (p. 123)

Nightingale believed that the only way nurses could overcome this oppressive barrier was through acute observation, careful documentation, and clear communication (Nightingale 1860/1969). Her emphasis on acute observation is reminiscent of the traditional healer's ability to see and smell illness. You repeatedly find in Nightingale's writings her belief that careful assessment is the foundation for all nursing care. Her words remind you that data alone are not sufficient; the nurse must critically collect information with one goal in mind. As Nightingale (1860/1969) wrote, "It must never be lost sight of what observation is for. It is not for the sake of piling up miscellaneous information or curious facts, but for the sake of saving life and increasing health and comfort" (p. 125).

Nightingale (1860/1969) believed that the abilities to observe and accurately sense shifts in patient status were unique attributes of the nurse. She provided the following example:

> *In all diseases it is important, but in diseases that do not run a distinct and fixed course, it is not only important, it is essential that the facts the nurse alone can observe should be accurately observed, and accurately reported. (p. 122)*

The ability to accurately observe is such an essential part of nursing that Nightingale suggested, "If you cannot get the habit of observation one way or other, you had better give up the being of a nurse, for it is not your calling, however kind and anxious you may be" (p. 113). Nightingale's words are a reminder for nurses today that computers and technology cannot be relied on to pick up the subtlest shifts in patient status. Only the skilled bedside nurse can sense and observe the earliest signs indicating the patient is in danger.

Nightingale's commitment to partnership is also evident in her relationship with the environment. However, this aspect of her healing philosophy receives little mention—perhaps because it challenges one of the domination system's core beliefs: that humans are above nature. (This matter is discussed further in Chapter 12 of this book.) Like ancient healers before her, Nightingale (1860/1969) understood that we are part of the web of life. She wrote:

> *It is often thought that medicine is the curative process. It is no such thing; medicine is the surgery of functions, as surgery is that of limbs and organs. Neither can do anything but remove obstructions; neither can cure, nature alone cures. Surgery removes the bullet out of the limb, which is an obstruction to cure, but nature heals the wound. So it is with medicine; the function of an organ becomes obstructed; medicine, so far as we know, assists nature to remove the obstruction, but does nothing more. And what nursing has to do in either case is to put the patient in the best condition for nature to act upon him. (p. 133)*

Nightingale's brilliance lay in her innate understanding that when nature and nurses collaborate, healing is possible.

Walt Whitman (1819-1892)

"A great poem is for ages and ages in common and for all degrees and complexions and all departments and sects and for a woman as much as a man and a man as much as a woman. A great poem is no finish to a man or a woman but rather a beginning."

–Walt Whitman (1855/2010, p. 44)

Many have claimed that Walt Whitman was the greatest U.S. poet. He may also have been one of the greatest U.S. nurses. Whitman is best known for his collection of poems titled *Leaves of Grass* (1855/2010), in which he praised the merits of equality and unity. His passion for life in all its diverse forms provides a stark contrast to the realities of the domination paradigm, especially as it became manifest in the American Civil War.

When news arrived that his brother had been wounded while fighting for the Union in the American Civil War, Whitman rushed to Washington, DC, to try to find him. Instead, he found his calling to care. The Civil War of 1861-1865 was the deadliest war for the United States. Nearly 620,000 people lost their lives, but only one third of the deaths were directly related to battle injuries; the rest were due to infections and disease including typhoid fever, diarrhea, and pneumonia (Coviello, as cited in Whitman, 2004).

While Whitman visited gravely ill soldiers, he kept copious notes of his impressions. He later published them as *Memoranda During the War* (1876/2004). He summarized:

During my past three years in Hospital, camp or field, I made over 600 visits or tours, and went, as I estimate, among 80,000 to 100,000 of the wounded and sick, as sustainer of spirit, and body in some degree, in time of need … I can say that in my ministerings,

I comprehended all who ever came in my way, Northern or Southern, and slighted none. It afforded me, too, the perusal of those subtlest, rarest, divinest moments of Humanity, laid bare in its inmost recesses, and of actual life and death, better than the finest, most labor'd narratives, histories, poems in the libraries. It arous'd and brought out and decided undream'd-of depths of emotion. (p. 101)

Through his writings, Whitman described the emotions and lived experience of nursing. He also demonstrated that his ability to listen to the stories of those in need became his greatest medicine.

Some Whitman scholars do not consider Whitman a nurse due to his gender and lack of formal training (Coviello, as cited in Whitman, 2004; Morris, 2000). Even Whitman himself referred to himself as a "volunteer." He manifested, however, the essence of bedside care, challenging the domination myth that care and nurturing are gender linked. Regarding the medicine of being present (Potter, 2013), Whitman wrote this:

I supply often to some of these dear suffering boys in my presence and magnetism that which doctors nor medicines nor skills nor any routine assistance can give …. I can testify that friendship has literally cured a fever, and the medicine of daily affection, a bad wound. (Whitman, as cited in Morris, 2000, p. 6)

In *Memoranda During the War* (1876/2004), Whitman describes giving paper and stamps to soldiers so they could contact their families and bringing them small candies and jams as reminders of home. He sat by the side of lonely soldiers, listened to their most intimate stories, and provided them companionship as they died. In addition, he provided physical care when necessary. His poem "The Wound-Dresser" captures the lived experience of many nurses who have performed this skill (an excerpt follows):

Bearing the bandages, water and sponge,
Straight and swift to my wounded I go,
Where they lie on the ground after the battle brought in,
Where the priceless blood reddens the grass the ground,

Or to the rows of the hospital tent, or under the roof'd hospital,
To the long rows of cots up and down each side I return,
To each and all one after another I draw near, not one do I miss,
An attendant follows holding a tray, he carries a refuse pail,
Soon to be fill'd with clotted rags and blood, emptied, and fill'd
*   again.*

I onward go, I stop,
With hinged knees and steady hand to dress wounds,
I am firm with each, the pangs are sharp yet unavoidable,
One turns to me his appealing eyes-poor boy! I never knew you,
Yet I think I could not refuse this moment to die for you, if that
*   would save you.*

3

On, I go, (open doors of time! Open hospital doors!)
*   The crush'd head I dress, (poor crazed hand tear not the bandage*
*   away,)*
*   The neck of the cavalry-man with the bullet through and through*
*   I examine,*
*   Hard the breathing rattles, quite glazed already the eye, yet life*
*   struggles hard,*
*   (Come sweet death! Be persuaded O beautiful death!*
*   In mercy come quickly.)*

From the stump of the arm, the amputated hand,
I undo the clotted lint, remove the slough, wash off the matter
*   and blood,*
Back on his pillow the soldier bends with curv'd neck and side-
*   falling head,*
His eyes are closed, his face is pale, he dares not look on the
*   bloody stump,*
And has not yet look'd on it.

I dress the wound in the side, deep, deep,
But a day or two more, for see the frame all wasted and sinking,
And the yellow-blue countenance see.

I dress the perforated shoulder, the foot with the bullet-wound,
Cleanse the one with a gnawing and putrid gangrene, so sickening,
    so offensive,
While the attendant stands behind aside me holding the tray and
    pail.

I am faithful, I do not give out,
The fractur'd thigh, the knee, the wound in the abdomen,
These and more I dress with impassive hand, (yet deep in my breast
    a fire, a burning flame).

                    –Walt Whitman (as cited in Morris, 2000, pp. 121-123)

Whitman's poems challenged the domination myth of the glory of war and conquest, while his presence challenged the domination myth that care and compassion are the exclusive province of women.

Finally, in *Leaves of Grass,* Whitman (1855/2010) rewove the threads of ancient healing wisdom and partnership into a message for future generations:

This is what you shall do: Love the Earth and sun and animals,
despise riches, give alms to everyone that asks, stand up for the
stupid and crazy, devote your income and labor to others, hate
tyrants, argue not concerning God, have patience and indulgence
toward the people, take off your hat to nothing known or
unknown or to any man or number of men, go freely with powerful
uneducated persons and with the young and with the mothers of
families, read these leaves in the open air every season of every year
of your life, re-examine all you have been told at school or church
or in any book, dismiss whatever insults your own soul. (p. 23)

Lillian Wald (1867-1940)

Few nurses capture the spirit of prevention better than Lillian Wald. Her experience as a hospital nurse led her to believe that suffering could be decreased, and perhaps even prevented, if people were informed about healthy living and disease prevention. In her book, *The House on Henry Street* (1915), Wald recounted the story of her initial experience in New York's impoverished East Side and her realization of the falseness of domination myths about "inferior" classes:

> *A little girl led me one drizzling March morning. She had told me of her sick mother, and gathering from her incoherent account that a child had been born, I caught up the paraphernalia of the bed-making lesson and carried it with me.... The child led me over broken roadways—there was no asphalt, although its use was well established in other parts of the city—over dirty mattresses and heaps of refuse... between reeking houses whose laden fire-escapes, useless for the intended purpose, bulged with household goods of every description .... Past evil-smelling, uncovered garbage-cans; and—perhaps worst of all, where so many little children played— past the trucks brought down from fastidious quarters.... The child led me on... to a rear tenement, by slimy steps whose accumulated dirt was augmented that day by the mud of the streets, and finally into the sick room. All the maladjustments of our social and economic relations seemed epitomized in this brief journey and what was found at the end of it. The family to which the child led me was neither criminal nor vicious...and although the sick woman lay on a wretched, unclean bed, soiled with a hemorrhage two days old, they were not degraded human beings, judged by any measure of moral values. (pp. 4-6)*

Wald (1915) referred to this incident as her "baptism of fire" (p. 7). It also provided the spark of inspiration that eventually gave birth to public health nursing and school nursing. Wald, along with nursing colleague Mary Brewster, determined that a settlement would provide the best way to facilitate community outreach. Wald (1915) wrote, "We were to live in the neighborhood as nurses, identify ourselves with it socially, and, in brief contribute to it our citizenship" (p. 8). Through the Henry Street Settlement, Wald and Brewster became part of the community they served. Their community partnership resulted in dramatic improvement of health outcomes. For example, in 1914, the four large New York hospitals cared for a combined total of 1,612 pneumonia patients, with a mortality rate for those patients of 31.2%. During the same time period, the Henry Street nurses cared for 3,535 cases of pneumonia with a mortality rate of 8.05% (p. 38).

Despite successes, Wald and her associates were not exempt from subjugation and oppression by the medical establishment. The mood and attitude toward nurses was reflected in a 1901 issue of the *Journal of the American Medical Association* that claimed "many doctors found that a nurse was often conceited and too unconscious of the due subordination she owes to the medical profession, of which she is sort of a useful parasite" (Walsh, as cited in Achterberg, 1990, p. 162). Given the health care culture of the early 1900s, Wald's autonomy was even more remarkable. Wald (1915) wrote:

> *The nurse should be as ready to respond to calls from the people themselves as to calls from physicians.... The new basis of the visiting-nurse service, which we thus inaugurated, reacted almost immediately upon the relationship of the nurse to the patient, reversing the position the nurse had formerly held. (pp. 27-28)*

Wald clearly grasped the harmful impact that systems of domination have on health and the power of partnership to both prevent illness and promote healing. Indeed, one of Wald's (1915) greatest legacies was to call nurses to confidently become true partners in healing. She wrote:

> *[The nurse is] enlisted in the crusade against disease and for the promotion of right living, beginning even before life itself is brought forth, through infancy into school life, on through adolescence, with its appeal to repair the omissions of the past. Her duties take her into factory and workshop, and she has identified herself with the movement against the premature employment of children, and for the protection of men and women who work that*

they may not risk health and life itself while earning their living....
Her contribution to human welfare, unified and harmonized with
those powers which aim at care and prevention rather than at
police power and punishment, forms part of the great policy of
bringing human beings to a higher level. (p. 60)

Wald made major contributions because she had the courage to defy
traditions of domination in order to reform inadequate systems of care. School
nurses, public health nurses, and home care nurses all owe this remarkable
woman a great debt of gratitude.

Margaret Sanger (1879-1966)

"A woman who behaves as a sexually and economically free person
is a threat to the entire social and economic fabric of a rigidly male-
dominated society. Such behavior cannot be countenanced lest the
entire social and economic system fall apart. Hence the 'necessity'
for the strongest social and religious condemnation and most
extreme punishment."

–Eisler (1987, p. 97)

Margaret Sanger challenged the domination system at an even more fundamental
level. She took on one of its chief modes of subjugating women: the control of
women's bodies (Eisler, 1995). Sanger displayed enormous courage in the face
of huge obstacles and harsh criticism. The following words of one German
physician epitomized the sentiment of many physicians at the time: "We will
never give over the control of our numbers to the women themselves. What, let
them control the future of the human race? ... We make the decisions, and they
must come to us" (as cited by Sanger, 1923/1971, p. 286).

Once she saw the horrible suffering of women related to lack of access to
contraception, Sanger asserted that women have the right to govern their own
sexuality and control their own role in conception. Her path included spending
time in jail because she refused to give up her fight for this fundamental right for
women (Sanger, 1923/1971). Sanger's conviction that access to contraception

is essential for the health of women and children was based on her experiences while nursing new mothers. In *Margaret Sanger: An Autobiography* (1923/1971), she wrote:

> *Always I was deeply affected by the trust patients, rich or poor, male or female, old or young, placed in their nurses.... Mothers asked me pathetically, plaintively, hopefully, "Miss Higgins, what should I do to not have another baby right away?" I was at a loss to answer their intimate questions, and passed them along to the doctor, who more often than not snorted, "She ought to be ashamed of herself to talk to a young girl about things like that." (p. 55)*

The turning point for Sanger came when she was called to provide home nursing care for Mrs. Sachs, a woman with septicemia related to a self-induced abortion. Desperation had led Mrs. Sachs to attempt to end her pregnancy because she knew her husband's meager salary would be incapable of feeding one more child. Several weeks later, when the doctor came to make his last home visit, Sanger informed him that Mrs. Sachs was concerned about having another baby.

> *"She may well be," replied the doctor, then he stood before her and said, "Any more such capers, young woman, and there'll be no need to send for me." "I know, doctor," she replied timidly, "but." And she hesitated as though it took all her courage to say it, "what can I do to prevent it?..." The doctor laughed good-naturedly. "You want to have your cake and eat it too, do you? Well it can't be done.... Tell Jake to sleep on the roof." (Sanger, 1923/1971, p. 92)*

Three months later Mrs. Sachs died from another abortion attempt.

This all too frequent tragedy made Sanger realize that most women in the United States did not know how to limit the size of their families. With adequate funds, some wealthy women could receive counseling, advice, and even skilled termination of pregnancies. But poor and middle-class women had access only to folk remedies and risky self-induced abortions. Observing that limited family incomes could not adequately support large families, Sanger concluded that lack of adequate contraceptive knowledge also put children at risk for illness and malnutrition. (Sanger, 1923/1971).

Sanger first attempted to write and publish articles about contraception options. After submitting one such article, she opened the newspaper eager to see her article "What Every Girl Should Know" in print. But instead of what she had written, she found "'What Every Girl Should Know: NOTHING!' By order of the Post Office Department" (Sanger, 1923/1971, p. 77). Sanger, however, was not deterred. She courageously refused to have her mission thwarted by censorship (Figure 5.1). Then she went even further.

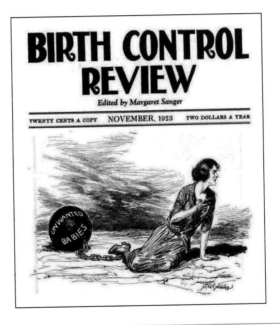

FIGURE 5.1 COVER OF BIRTH CONTROL REVIEW, NOVEMBER, 1923.

On October 16, 1916, Sanger opened the first clinic in the United States where women could come for classes and be informed about contraception options, or what she termed "birth control." It did not take long for the domination system to respond: Sanger was arrested and her clinic closed.

The following scene, described by Sanger, illustrates the desperation of women at the time:

Two uniformed policemen came for me... as we started I heard a scream from a woman who had just come around the corner on her way to the clinic. She abandoned her baby carriage, rushed through the crowd, and cried, "Come back! Come back and save me!" (Sanger, 1923/1971, pp. 222-223)

Women in the United States today can access information about contraception thanks to nurse Margaret Sanger. She not only had the courage to defy oppressive laws that enforced a centuries-old system that controlled women's bodies, she had the vision and determination to create ways for women to avoid the terrible suffering this control caused them and their families. Later, her "birth control clinics" came to be known as Planned Parenthood (Sanger, 1923/1971).

Mary Breckinridge (1881-1965)

Mary Breckinridge was born into a family with power, prestige, and great land holdings. She was not content, however, with the low expectations for women. Few women went to college, and those who did frequently married, leaving any dreams of an independent profession behind (Breckinridge, 1952).

Breckinridge experienced many personal losses before she started her nursing work. Her first husband died suddenly, she lost a daughter in a stillbirth, her beloved son Breckie died at age 4, and this was followed closely by a divorce from her second husband. These losses fueled her drive to serve (Breckinridge, 1952).

Breckinridge was passionate about children and felt there was no greater calling than to work to raise the status of children. In *Wide Neighborhoods: A Story of the Frontier Nursing Service,* Breckinridge (1952) wrote:

Nurse-midwifery is the logical response to the needs of the child in rural America.... Work for children should begin before they are born, should carry them through their greatest hazard, which is childbirth, and should be most intensive during their first six years of life. These are the formative years—whether for their bodies, their minds, or their loving hearts. (p. 111)

At that time, nursing and midwifery were rarely integrated. For example, French midwives were not nurses, U.S. nurses were not midwives, and only British nurses were both. Breckinridge traveled to England, where she studied and became a Certified English Nurse Midwife. From there she ventured to Scotland and studied the effective Highlands and Islands Medical and Nursing Service.

Upon her return to the United States, Breckinridge began her life's work, establishing the Frontier Nursing Service. She chose Kentucky for its inaccessibility, believing that if her model worked there it could work anywhere. In the early 1920s, the remote mountain regions of eastern Kentucky had few roads and even fewer physicians. Breckinridge realized that if people were to receive adequate health care, the care had to be brought to them; this meant that nurses in the Frontier Nursing Service traveled miles and miles on horseback to visit families in need.

The first remote Frontier Nursing Service clinic opened in 1925, and eventually Breckinridge created an entire system of rural clinics so each territory had access to nursing services. A nurse midwife who taught health classes and made rounds to clients on horseback staffed each clinic. Breckinridge (1952) described her experience:

As I rode from place to place I gave such nursing care as I could to the sick people I met, especially the babies.... Sometimes I was able to hand a pink baby back to a mother who had given me a blue one. When I had done all I could for the child, I talked with its mother, and with the other mothers, who had gathered around me, not only about how to take care of the sick babies, but how to feed all the second summer babies in such a way as to keep them well. It was because my nursing skill helped the sick babies that the mothers welcomed my suggestions. (pp. 164-165)

Community collaboration was a hallmark of the Frontier Nursing Service.

Breckinridge's (1952) philosophy of working through the community rather than for the community was tremendously successful. Very little is accomplished by entering a community and telling people how things must be done—Breckinridge instead worked in partnership with the community. Community members helped plan and build their own clinics, and they were allowed to pay for services any way they could. As Breckinridge reported:

> There was so little "cash money" in the mountains for years after we started our work that our five-dollar midwifery fee (which included complete care in childbirth, prenatal care, and nursing visits for ten days after the baby was born) was rarely paid in money. In lieu of this fee, we accepted quilted "kivers" from the women, homemade split-bottomed chairs from their husbands, food from those who had a small surplus, and the husband's labor in mending fences and whitewashing barns. (p. 202)

This exchange of goods for services is reminiscent of ancient partnership communities where the community cared for the healer in exchange for the healer's skills.

Like other nursing visionaries, Breckinridge understood that statistics could provide important support for new models of care. After Breckinridge delivered Frontier Nursing Service data to the Metropolitan Life Insurance Company, the company representative concluded the following:

> If such a service was available to the women of the country generally, there would be a saving of 10,000 mothers' lives a year in the United States, there would be 30,000 less stillbirths and 30,000 children alive at the end of the first month of life. (Breckinridge, 1952, p. 312)

Breckinridge and her nurses on horseback successfully demonstrated the effectiveness of partnership-based community nursing care.

Mamie Odessa Hale (1911-1979)

Though she did not write an autobiography and is not well known outside Arkansas, Mamie Odessa Hale made important contributions as a nurse. In the 1930s and 1940s, rural Arkansas Blacks were severely impoverished and subjugated. Racial discrimination created major health disparities, there were very few African-American physicians, and most Blacks could not afford either health care or transportation to hospitals. Statistics revealed the depth of these health care disparities: "In 1941 there were 142 deaths in childbirth among black women, of which 107 could have been avoided" (Belle, 1993, p. 127). The maternal and infant mortality rates were also nearly twice as high in Blacks as in whites.

At that time, 75% of Blacks in Arkansas utilized *granny midwives* for their deliveries: women mostly aged 60 to 80 who were well-respected folk healers without any formal training. Belle (1993) reported that three-quarters of the granny midwives were illiterate, which proved particularly challenging when it came to completing birth certificates. This was significant because every live birth that went unreported meant federal funding would not be awarded to the state.

After Mamie Odessa Hale graduated from the Tuskegee School of Nurse-Midwifery, she was hired by the Arkansas State Board of Health to work with the granny midwives (Figure 5.2). She designed an 8–12 week training for them that culminated with state certification. Several elements of Hale's training course displayed partnership values (Belle, 1993):

- The sessions were held in the locations most accessible for the granny midwives.

- Hale allowed the midwives to be assisted by community members when filling out birth certificates.

- Theory content was delivered in the form of movies and demonstrations, so literacy was not required.

- Hale empowered the midwives to limit their caseloads to safe levels.

- Granny midwives "attributed their position of midwife to a 'divine call-ing.' Nurse Hale encouraged this belief by organizing meetings around a religious theme, opening them with hymn singing and prayer" (Belle, 1993, p. 161).

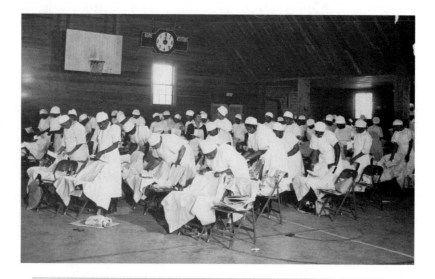

FIGURE 5.2 MAMIE ODESSA HALE TEACHING A CLASS OF COMMUNITY MIDWIVES. HALE IS IN THE CENTER OF THE PHOTO IN A BLACK DRESS AND APRON.
Courtesy of the UAMS Library's Historical Research Center

Hale demonstrated deep respect for the people she served and managed to walk the fine line between ushering in changes that would improve public health and demanding changes that would harm the community's culture.

Being Black herself, Hale (1948) was very aware of racial tensions and forces of oppression. Her approach was to find ways to empower those who were subjugated. She wrote:

About three-fourths of the midwives in the Delta area live on plantations; so during the series of classes the midwife sometimes has difficulty in convincing her "boss man" that it is necessary to be away.... The nurse-midwife gets the names of all plantation owners in the county, every physician, teacher, registrar of vital statistics, and all the key people in the county. Then each receives a letter of invitation from the county health department. (p. 53)

In this way Hale built coalitions to support the granny midwives during their training. She used hierarchies of actualization to limit the power and control of domination.

The graduation ceremony exemplified other aspects of partnership. Hale (1948) wrote that as she spoke to the community, she stressed the qualifications of a good midwife and the responsibility midwives and communities held for each other—she built empowering relationships instead of hierarchies of domination. For her, the primary goal of a formal graduation ceremony was to increase the prestige of the granny midwives so families would seek earlier prenatal care.

Both quantitative and qualitative data demonstrated the effectiveness of Hale's approach. Belle (1993) summarizes Hale's contributions:

The number of black deaths due to pregnancy and childbirth fell from 128 in 1930 to 43 in 1950. These accomplishments speak highly of the work of Nurse Mamie Hale for she convinced granny midwives to accept the idea that State Health Department classes were important and useful. She found ways to instruct midwives despite their advanced ages, superstitious beliefs, and widespread illiteracy. (p. 166)

Hale worked "with" the people instead of "above" them. She began with what they knew, respected them for their accomplishments, did not force but rather invited change, and ultimately raised the status of traditional healers.

Sister Elizabeth Kenny (1880-1952)

Few nursing stories demonstrate the tension between the domination and partnership paradigms better than the story of Sister Elizabeth Kenny. Kenny grew up in Australia, trained as a nurse, and started her career as a district (community) nurse. During World War I, she served with the Australian Imperial Forces where she received a promotion from staff nurse to sister, a rank similar to first lieutenant in the Army (Kenny & Ostenso, 1943). Kenny's most challenging battles were not on the battlefield, however—they were fought in hospitals, the halls of government, and the press.

The story begins with Kenny's younger brother Bill, who was born with extremely weak muscles that made him tire easily and require "piggy-back" rides to school. In an attempt to assist her brother, Kenny read every book on muscle anatomy that she could lay her hands on, including medical textbooks loaned by their family physician. This early interest in service led her to contemplate missionary work, where she was informed a nursing background would prove invaluable (Kenny & Ostenso, 1943). Kenny started her work as a visiting nurse in the Australian bush; there she realized her true calling and began her life work.

Kenny was only 23 years old when she first encountered infantile paralysis, which is now called *poliomyelitis*. In her autobiography *And They Shall Walk* (Kenny & Ostenso, 1943), Kenny describes in detail her first exposure to this devastating disease:

> *She lay upon a cot in the most alarming attitude. One knee was drawn up towards the face and the other foot was pointed downwards. The little heel was twisted and turned outward, or abducted. One arm lay with flexed elbow across the chest. Any attempt to straighten a member caused the child extreme pain. The little golden-haired girl who had gladdened my former stay in this humble home was indeed very sick, and with an ailment that was unknown to me. For the moment, I felt beaten, since I did not know what to do until I could get the necessary medical advice.* (p. 23)

Kenny quickly rode her horse to a telegraph office miles away and sent a telegram to the nearest physician. While she waited for a response, another frantic rancher showed up and reported that two of his kids "had been taken with what he called the 'cow disease' and neither of them could stand or walk"

(p. 23). The medical response to her question arrived via a telegram that simply said, "Infantile Paralysis. No known treatment. Do the best you can with the symptoms presenting themselves" (Kenny & Ostenso, 1943, p. 23). These words proved prophetic; Kenny addressed the symptoms, and in doing so, she eventually changed the world.

Kenny returned to the little hut, and after saying a prayer for divine guidance, she attempted to relieve the symptoms. She noted that the child tried to protect the severely contracted muscles from any stretching because any amount of stretching increased her pain. Kenny's knowledge of muscle anatomy informed her that deformity could possibly result if the contractures were not relieved. She filled a bag with hot salt and applied it to the affected limb, but her first attempt at pain relief was unsuccessful. Then she tried poultices made with linseed meal, but these were too heavy. Eventually, in desperation, she tore a wool blanket into strips, soaked the strips in boiling water, and gently wrapped them around the contracted limbs. Kenny wrote:

> *The whimpering of the child ceased almost immediately …. After a short while, however, the little slumberer awoke fretfully and cried out, "I want them rags that wells my legs!" And so the little girl of the Australian bushland unknowingly spoke approval of a treatment that was one day to become the subject of much heated debate among the learned members of the medical world. (Kenny & Ostenso, 1943, pp. 24-25)*

Despite the effectiveness of Kenny's method of treating infantile paralysis, those who embraced the domination paradigm did all they possibly could to prevent this knowledge from spreading (Kenny & Ostenso, 1943). Hierarchies of domination only allow one-way communication. Those people seen as having a lower rank are forbidden from challenging the decisions of those with higher rank. Women, and therefore most nurses, are forbidden from voicing their views and opinions, especially if they contradict the opinions and explanations of males or physicians. Systems of domination support and permit only one form of knowledge, thereby thwarting interprofessional practice, true patient- and family-centered care, and innovation to promote effective health care models.

For many years Kenny operated a small clinic where people brought their paralyzed children for treatments. Earlier in her career, she designed and patented an ambulance stretcher for shock victims; the royalties she received from the "Sylvia Stretcher" allowed her to provide therapies to paralyzed children free of charge. Of this time period, Kenny wrote:

> *As time passed, one sad-hearted mother after another brought her child to the little cottage hospital and took them home again with no visible disability. But the medical men withheld their recognition. The record of my work was written only in the hearts of the people. (Kenny & Ostenso, 1943, p. 32)*

Eventually, so many people had benefited from Kenny's method that the medical community could no longer ignore her. Kenny's notoriety led to an invitation to speak before a medical audience. Kenny wrote:

> *I described the isolation of the Australian bush country where I had first encountered the disease. There were no scientific research workers, no well-equipped laboratory, not even a cottage hospital. There was only a cot and a tortured child—and a desire to relieve the child's pain by any means possible. It would not have occurred to me to apply splints. I saw the limbs being pulled out of shape— not as was thought by the medical world, by strong muscles pulling weak ones, but by painful spasmodic contractions of affected muscles. I saw a painful muscle condition that meant agony for the child. And I treated only what I saw. (Kenny & Ostenso, 1943, p. 230)*

Kenny proposed the following:

> *The true symptoms of infantile paralysis were not the symptoms that had been accepted by the medical profession throughout the world. I have described the true symptoms as "opposite" to those that have been recognized by orthodox practitioners.... The old theory that deformities were caused by "strong muscles pulling weak muscles" was a fallacy. Deformities are caused by spasm in the affected muscles. By splinting and other means of*

immobilization, the orthodox treatment sought to forestall or to correct deformities in the acute stage. I discarded the procedure as being not only unnecessary and painful to the patient, but as being definitely damaging and frequently disastrous in its effects.... For generations, in short, orthodoxy had been treating for symptoms that did not exist. (p. 241)

The story of Kenny's method for treating infantile paralysis is really a story of the power of entrenched paradigms or belief systems.

The fact that Kenny, a nurse, would dare to question established beliefs and orthodox treatment brought a swift and harsh response by the medical system. Kenny later concluded:

I was wholly unprepared for the extraordinary attitude of the medical world in its readiness to condemn anything that smacked of reform or that ran contrary to approved methods of practice. I can understand how necessary it may be that new methods should be examined critically and that all the evidence must be carefully weighed before approval can be given. But I have also wondered how many promising discoveries have been consigned to oblivion without being given an opportunity to prove their worth. (Kenny & Ostenso, 1943, p. 2)

Kenny's autobiography (Kenny & Ostenso, 1943) included numerous stories about her marginalization and the subjugation of her method for treating infantile paralysis. Kenny's experiences included detractors claiming the children she helped did not truly have infantile paralysis. She encountered anger because she had not used proper channels to report her work to leading experts. Physicians claimed they had toured her clinic and evaluated her work when they had done no such thing. One physician went so far as to steal the only copy of a book Kenny was writing about her method so he could open a clinic under his own control.

Kenny and Ostenso (1943) told the story about a doctor who brought his own son to see Kenny because all other methods of treating the son's infantile paralysis had failed. After the treatments were successful, the grateful father was willing to tell his story to the newspapers, but unwilling to discuss the success of the case with his medical peers. In addition, Kenny reported another doctor "with his own theories and books about infantile paralysis said, 'I should be relieved of any association with the work of the clinic because of the bad effect my presence had on the honorary medical staff'" (Kenny & Ostenso, 1943, p. 183). One doctor even went so far as to say, "Doctors are not going to be taught by a nurse. Surely you do not think you can teach anything to the commission" (Kenny & Ostenso, 1943, p. 126). Fortunately, Sister Elizabeth Kenny did not let the domination paradigm triumph.

In Minneapolis, Minnesota, in the United States, Kenny found medical practitioners open to new ways of thinking. She informed them that in order to learn her method, they would have to unlearn everything they thought they knew to be true about infantile paralysis. She invited them to think of infantile paralysis as a new disease that had a remarkably effective treatment (Kenny & Ostenso, 1943).

One particular group of skeptical physicians visited her, and all 10 certified that the child before them was completely paralyzed and beyond hope. Kenny wrote:

> *I disagreed and stepped forward. Again, as I had done in my own wild out-back of Australia over thirty years before, I taught the muscle what to do, gave back to it its motor pattern, and then linked it up with the brain path. Full use of the muscle was restored in less than twenty seconds. (Kenny & Ostenso, 1943, p. 255)*

Needless to say, these skeptics were convinced.

Minnesota's physicians opened their minds so they could objectively analyze data on Kenny's patients. While Australia's medical reports stated, "Her abandonment of immobilization is a grievous error and fraught with great danger—especially on young children who cannot co-operate in reeducation" (Kenny & Ostenso, 1943, p. 225), the University of Minnesota's physicians were willing to shift their paradigm. They wrote, "We have no hesitation in saying this method will form the basis of all future treatment .... Absolutely no deformities have materialized.... They were more limber than they were before they had the disease" (p. 225).

Being open to the knowledge of other professions, being able to examine previous assumptions, and being willing to work interprofessionally made it possible for thousands of children with polio to eventually walk without braces. Once Kenny's method received the backing of a prestigious research university, her treatments were taught to nurses, therapists, and parents around the country. A grateful nation bestowed on Kenny numerous honors including Humanitarian Medals, an honorary degree of doctor of science, and an invitation to meet President Franklin Delano Roosevelt, himself a victim of polio (Kenny & Ostenso, 1943).

This courageous outback nurse changed the world by partnering with each patient's symptoms to alleviate his or her suffering. Kenny closed her autobiography with a message for future generations:

> To the men and women of the future, therefore I give freely what I have done. May they and the generations to come, equipped with all that modern science can provide, dedicate the labor of their hands and the devotion of their hearts to the end that healing may be brought to the suffering children of every land, every creed, and of every race. (Kenny & Ostenso, 1943, p. 272)

Conclusion

As you have seen, underlying recorded history has been the tension between two basic models of social organization. The domination model consists of hierarchies of domination, with the subjugation of women and other marginalized groups; the partnership model is based on egalitarianism and hierarchies of actualization where power is used to empower rather than disempower (Eisler, 1987, 1995, 2007).

The stories in this chapter show that many nurses have embraced partnership. They partnered with nature and the web of life. They partnered with their calling. They were partners with patients at the bedside and in communities. And they recognized and collaborated with the innate healing wisdom of the human body. These nurses persevered, even though under the domination paradigm it could be dangerous to live according to principles of partnership. Nurses who challenged domination thinking were extremely courageous. Despite personal risk, they often worked autonomously to develop effective models of care, serving patients with unmet needs and underserved communities.

We need to hear their stories and retell them to our children and our children's children. We need to add our own stories, too, for we are partners in healing. The story of nursing has just begun.

TABLE 5.1 Historic Nurses and What Their Stories Tell Us

NURSE	PARTNERSHIP PRINCIPLE ILLUSTRATED
Mary Seacole	Democratic and economically equitable structure of linking and hierarchies of actualization in both family and state
	Conflict creatively used to arrive at solutions
Florence Nightingale	Equal valuing of the male and female halves of humanity
	Empathic, mutually beneficial, and caring relations are considered moral and desirable
Walt Whitman	Fluid gender roles with high valuing of empathy, caring, caregiving, and nonviolence
	Leadership based on power to (woman or man who nurtures and supports productivity and creativity) and/or power with (encourages and participates in teamwork)
Lillian Wald	Democratic and economically equitable structure of linking
	High valuing of empathy, caring, caregiving, and non-violence in both women and men, as well as in social and economic policy

NURSE	PARTNERSHIP PRINCIPLE ILLUSTRATED
	Conflict creatively used to arrive at solutions
	Leadership based on power to (woman or man who nurtures and supports productivity and creativity) and/or power with (encourages and participates in teamwork)
	Hierarchies of actualization: fluid hierarchies that empower others for optimal functioning
Margaret Sanger	Equal valuing of the male and female halves of humanity
	Democratic and economically equitable structure of linking and hierarchies of actualization in both family and state
	Conflict creatively used to arrive at solutions
	Leadership based on power to (woman or man who nurtures and supports productivity and creativity) and/or power with (encourages and participates in teamwork)
Mary Breckinridge	Democratic and economically equitable structure of linking
	Give high value to empathic, mutually beneficial, and caring relations, which are considered moral and desirable
	Trust and reciprocity-based cooperation
	Leadership based on power to (woman or man who nurtures and supports productivity and creativity) and/or power with (encourages and participates in teamwork)
	Hierarchies of actualization: fluid hierarchies that empower others for optimal functioning
Mamie Odessa Hale	Emphasis on democratic and equitable health care
	Mutual respect and trust with a low degree of fear, abuse, and violence
	Trust and reciprocity-based cooperation

continues

TABLE 5.1 Continued

NURSE	PARTNERSHIP PRINCIPLE ILLUSTRATED
	Conflict creatively used to arrive at solutions
	Leadership based on power to (woman or man who nurtures and supports productivity and creativity) and/or power with (encourages and participates in teamwork)
	Hierarchies of actualization: fluid hierarchies that empower others for optimal functioning
Sister Elizabeth Kenny	Equal valuing of the male and female halves of humanity
	Democratic and economically equitable structure of linking and hierarchies of actualization in both family and state
	Conflict creatively used to arrive at solutions
	Hierarchies of actualization: fluid hierarchies that empower others for optimal functioning

Adapted from Riane Eisler, The Power of Partnership *(2002). See also Table 3.1 in this book.*

References

Achterberg, J. (1990). *Woman as healer.* Boston, MA: Shambhala.

Belle, P. (1993). "Making do" with the midwife: Arkansas's Mamie O. Hale in the 1940s. *Nursing History Review, 1,* 155-169.

Bostridge, M. (2008). *Florence Nightingale: The making of an icon.* New York, NY: Farrar, Straus, and Giroux.

Breckinridge, M. (1952). *Wide neighborhoods: A story of the Frontier Nursing Service.* Lexington, KY: University Press of Kentucky.

Eisler, R. (1987). *The chalice and the blade: Our history, our future.* San Francisco, CA: Harper & Row.

Eisler, R. (1995). *Sacred pleasure: Sex, myth, and the politics of the body.* San Francisco, CA: HarperCollins.

Eisler, R. (2002). *The power of partnership.* Novato, CA: New World Library.

Eisler, R. (2007). *Real wealth of nations: Creating a caring economics.* San Francisco, CA: Berrett-Koehler.

Hale, M. O. (1948). Arkansas midwives have all-day graduation exercises. *The Child, 13*(4), 53-54.

Kenny, E., & M. Ostenso. (1943). *And they shall walk.* New York, NY: Dodd, Mead, & Company.

Lopez, B. (1990). *Crow and weasel.* New York, NY: North Point Press.

Morris, R. (2000). *The better angel: Walt Whitman in the Civil War.* Oxford, UK: Oxford University Press.

Nightingale, F. (1969). *Notes on nursing: What it is and what it is not.* New York, NY: Dover. (Original work published 1860)

Potter, T. M. (2010). Reconstructing a new story of nursing: Critical analysis of nursing textbooks using Riane Eisler's partnership paradigm. *Dissertation Abstracts International, 72*(05), 3447086.

Potter, T. M. (2013). *The BASE of nursing.* Unpublished manuscript, School of Nursing, University of Minnesota, United States of America.

Rushdie, S. (1988). *The satanic verses.* New York, NY: Picador.

Sanger, M. (1971). *Margaret Sanger: An autobiography.* New York, NY: Dover. (Original work published 1923)

Seacole, M. (2005). *Wonderful adventures of Mrs. Seacole in many lands.* New York, NY: Penguin Books. (Original work published 1857)

Wald, L. (1915). *The house on Henry Street.* New York, NY: Henry Holt.

Whitman, W. (2004). *Memoranda during the war.* P. Coviello (Ed.). New York, NY: Oxford University Press. (Original work published 1876)

Whitman, W. (2010). *Leaves of grass.* L. Ross (Ed.). New York, NY: Sterling Innovation. (Original work published 1855)

Part III
A Systems Approach to Partnership-Based Nursing

"We need to be prepared to question every single aspect of the old paradigm. Eventually we will not need to throw everything away, but before we know that, we need to be willing to question everything... about the very foundations of our modern, scientific, industrial, growth-oriented, materialistic worldview and way of life."

–Fritjof Capra in The Web of Life:
A New Understanding of Living Systems, *1996, p. 8*

Health care is a complex system. Reforming health care will therefore require a systematic approach, or, in Capra's words, questioning "every single aspect of the old paradigm." Three objectives must be accomplished to facilitate nursing's shift to a partnership paradigm:

- First, harmful assumptions and self-limiting perceptions of the domination story must be revealed. (You read about this in Chapter 3.)

- Second, a partnership story must be told that includes a reconstructed recorded history and exemplars of partnership nursing. (Chapters 4 and 5 covered this story.)

- The final objective is to teach nurses how to serve collaboratively with clients, communities, other care providers, and the entire planetary eco-system.

This last objective is addressed in the seven chapters that follow (**Chapters 6 through 12**). Each of these chapters follows a similar template:

- Discussing ongoing domination challenges

- Describing an alternative partnership approach

- Offering a current partnership-based exemplar

The entire nursing system is examined from the partnership perspective, starting with nursing education, moving to nursing's relationships with stakeholders, and concluding with the role nursing can play in fostering a partnership-based society.

Our objective is not to exhaust the dialogue, but to start the conversation. Our hope is that you will begin recognizing threads of domination when they occur in all the various levels of health care today. Once you recognize them, you can challenge these threads and replace them with a partnership approach. Being fully conscious of the domination/partnership continuum allows you to choose the health care system you want for the future, and to live and work in such a way that it comes to pass.

Chapter 6
Transforming Nursing Education With Partnership

"Classroom teachers must step out from behind the screen full of slides and engage students in clinic-like learning experiences that ask them to learn to use knowledge and practice thinking in changing situations, always for the good of the patient."
–Benner, Sutphen, Leonard, and Day, 2010, p. 14

The Institute of Medicine (IOM, 2010) acknowledges that nurses are positioned to be both leaders of change and advocates for advancing health. Three factors suggest that we are today in a unique position to do this:

- Nursing has over 19 million members worldwide, outnumbering physicians two to one, thereby being the largest health care profession worldwide (World Health Organization [WHO], 2011).

- By definition, the nursing profession is focused on both prevention and quality care, and nurses have steadily advocated for safe environments and effective health care policy (International Council of Nurses [ICN], 2010).

- In the United States, for the 11th year in a row, nurses have topped the list when the Gallup poll asked citizens to rate the honesty and ethical standards of people in different fields (Robert Wood Johnson Foundation, 2012).

Given their important role, their numbers, and society's positive perception of nurses, the nursing profession has tremendous potential to impact health care policy and delivery. But there are challenges.

Identifying Patterns of Domination

An effective and sustainable health care system requires that nurses be educated for interprofessional practice and other partnership-based relationships. Before describing the characteristics of *partnership education*, however, you should know how to identify domination elements that still persist. As you will see in this chapter, these include:

- Pedagogies (teaching philosophies) based on domination values

- Rigid professional hierarchies and silos

- Hierarchies of nursing knowledge and evidence

Domination Pedagogies

Nurse educators can unwittingly reinforce the domination paradigm with the way they treat students. Writing about partnership in nursing education, Potter (2012a) shared the following personal experience:

I left full-time practice in the field because of a desire to help shape the next generation of nurses. With my newly awarded master of science in nursing, I started teaching theory and clinical courses at a local college. I love bedside nursing and was eager to share the magic of our profession with novices. On my first day of clinicals, I was surprised to find the units empty—not a student in sight. Strange! We all started the day together—where did they all go? Finally, I cornered one student who reported in a shaky voice, "We always run and hide when we see an instructor approaching. Who wants to be treated poorly?" (p. 47)

After this incident, Potter asked colleagues and practicing nurses about their experiences. Many recalled having at least one nursing instructor who made them question their abilities and even doubt their own observations.

Studies have documented the outcome of these kinds of negative experiences. For example, in the United Kingdom, Randle (2003) studied the impact nursing education had on the self-esteem of nursing students in a 3-year program. She reported:

Although the majority of students start their nurse training with normal self-esteem, they leave the course with below average self-esteem. In particular, not only did their overall self-esteem decrease dramatically, but also at the same time self-satisfaction, family, personal and social components of their self-esteem decreased. (p. 143)

How will nurses learn autonomy if they cannot trust their own observations? How can they become full partners in interprofessional education (IPE) teams if their self-esteem is weak? Clearly the teaching style of all nurse educators must shift from domination to partnership.

Domination Reinforced Through Silos and Professional Hierarchies

Nursing education also supports the domination paradigm when it either consciously or unconsciously maintains rigid silos or reinforces hierarchies within the health care professions. Patricia Benner, best known for her works *From Novice to Expert: Excellence and Power in Clinical Nursing Practice* (1984) and *Educating Nurses: A Call for Radical Transformation* (Benner, Sutphen, Leonard, & Day, 2010), forcefully challenges these hierarchies and silos. She notes that "IPE seeks to solve the disparate and hierarchical expectations of professional performance for the sake of patients and population health" (Benner, 2012, p. 3). In short, Benner urges the culture to move beyond professional hierarchies to interprofessional partnership-based nursing education.

The Lancet Commission report "Health Professionals for a New Century: Transforming Education to Strengthen Health Systems in an Interdependent World" (Frenk et al., 2010) also calls for major education reform in health care. The authors state that instructional reforms need to "promote interprofessional and transprofessional education that breaks down professional silos while enhancing collaborative and non-hierarchical relationships in effective teams" (Frenk et al., 2010, p. 1924).

Domination Through Hierarchies of Knowledge and Evidence

In 1972, British epidemiologist Archie Cochrane published *Effectiveness and Efficiency: Random Reflections on Health Services*. The principles in his book radically transformed health care practice.

Recognizing the chronic scarcity of health care resources, Cochrane declared that resources "should be used to provide equitably those forms of health care which had been shown in properly designed evaluations to be effective" (Cochrane Collaboration, n.d.a, "Background" section). In other words, given limited resources, the most just and effective approach to health resource allocation is to make treatments and interventions known to be efficacious available to all people.

Cochrane coined the term *evidence-based health care*, which he defined as:

The conscientious use of current best evidence in making decisions about the care of individual patients or the delivery of health services. Current best evidence is up-to-date information from relevant, valid research about the effects of different forms of health care, the potential for harm from exposure to particular agents, the accuracy of diagnostic tests, and the predictive power of prognostic factors. (Cochrane Collection, n.d.b, "Evidence-based health care" section)

Based on Cochrane's vision, the Cochrane Collaboration was launched. This nonprofit organization produces systematic reviews of research, which are widely considered the standard for evidence-based health care.

Even though randomized controlled trials (RCTs) became Cochrane's gold standard for determining the most reliable form of evidence, it is noteworthy that this important organization explicitly recognizes the importance of partnership, as expressed in this statement: "The Collaboration believes that effective health care is created through equal partnerships between researcher, provider, practitioner and patient" (Cochrane Collaboration, n.d.c, "About us" section).

The heavy emphasis on RCTs has had unintended consequences that were not foreseen by Cochrane. The trend towards a hierarchy of evidence marginalizes knowledge from other fields and consequently perpetuates patterns of domination. This problem is particularly acute in the use of what today is called *evidence-based medicine*. This term has led to the privileging of quantifiable data over the qualitative information so vital for accurate diagnosis and treatment. How did this happen?

Even though biomedicine has long been based on the scientific method, the term *evidence-based medicine* (EBM) began to appear in the literature in the 1990s when it was officially defined by Dr. David Sackett of Canada (Claridge & Fabian, 2005). After that, EBM rapidly became the practice paradigm for physicians and, subsequently, nurses. This meant that the focus was more on quantitative data, and more specifically on data that can be reproduced in similar experiments—especially randomized controlled studies.

As a result, so-called *hierarchies of evidence* today rank quantitative studies over qualitative studies. In an article designed to teach nonresearchers how to find and value research, Greenhalgh (1997) summarized this commonly accepted hierarchy of evidence as follows:

1. Systematic reviews and meta-analyses

2. Randomized controlled trials with definitive results (confidence intervals that do not overlap the threshold clinically significant effect)

3. Randomized controlled trials with nondefinitive results (a point estimate that suggests a clinically significant effect but with confidence intervals overlapping the threshold for this effect)

4. Cohort studies

5. Case-control studies

6. Cross-sectional surveys

7. Case reports (p. 246)

Not only does this hierarchy of evidence privilege some sources of knowledge over others, but it has resulted in narrative studies often being dismissed as failing the generalizability test of true evidence. And this continues to be the case—even though Greenhalgh (1999) strongly defends the importance of narrative-based practice in medicine. Indeed, she advocates that both kinds of evidence be given equal weight when she writes:

> *Appreciating the narrative nature of illness experience and the intuitive and subjective aspects of clinical method does not require us to reject the principles of evidence based medicine. Nor does such an approach demand an inversion of the hierarchy of evidence so that personal anecdote carries more weight in decision making than the randomized controlled trial. Far from obviating the need for subjectivity in the clinical encounter, genuine evidence based practice actually presupposes an interpretive paradigm in which the patient experiences illness in a unique and contextual way. Furthermore, it is only within such an interpretive paradigm that a clinician can meaningfully draw on all aspects of evidence—his or her own case based experience, the patient's individual and cultural perspectives, and the results of rigorous clinical research trials and observational studies—to reach an integrated clinical judgment. (Greenhalgh, 1999, p. 318)*

Unfortunately, Greenhalgh's philosophy of balance and integration (which aligns with the BASE of Nursing described in Chapter 1) still has not gained prominence in health care education. Nor is that all. In nursing education today, much of the curriculum is focused on the development and use of randomized controlled trial (RCT) data, with very little time spent on developing skills that elicit narrative evidence.

And again this persists—even though it goes against the philosophy of David Sackett himself, the physician and educator who, as mentioned earlier, introduced the term *evidence-based medicine* (EBM). For example, when responding to earlier critiques of his work, Sackett, Rosenberg, Muir Gray, Haynes, and Richardson (1996) wrote:

> *Evidence based medicine is the conscientious, explicit, and judicious use of current best evidence in making decisions about the care of individual patients. The practice of evidence based medicine means integrating individual clinical expertise with the best available external clinical evidence from systematic research.* (p. 71)

Sackett and his colleagues also highlight two other important aspects of the initial evidence-based medicine theory: the role of patients and respect for diverse sources of knowledge.

Sackett et al. (1996) place the patient at the center of both clinical expertise and external clinical evidence. They explicitly state that clinical expertise includes "thoughtful identification and compassionate use of individual patients' predicaments, rights, and preferences in making clinical decisions about their care" (p. 71). In their article, the authors also make it very clear that neither clinical expertise nor best external evidence alone is sufficient. Best practice requires the full utilization of both sources of knowledge. Sackett et al. (1996) summarize the necessary balance of sources of knowledge as follows: "Without clinical expertise, practice risks becoming tyrannized... without current best evidence, practice risks becoming rapidly out of date, to the detriment of patients" (p. 72).

Nonetheless, a hierarchy of evidence still dominates biomedicine. Even though Sackett et al. (1996) call for partnerships between providers and patients and for valuing both clinical expertise and external clinical evidence, rigid ranking and *hierarchies of domination* (Eisler, 2002) continue within many health care systems today. As Greenhalgh (1997) points out, case reports and clinical experiences still hold the lowest ranking in accepted hierarchies of evidence.

Rolfe and Gardner (2005) also criticize this form of domination within nursing research. They describe a system that marginalizes reflective practice and qualitative methodologies because they are considered "soft research," while emphasizing the importance of "hard research" generated through randomized controlled tests. These authors directly challenge this hierarchy: "We believe that the practice of nursing is fundamentally different from the practice of medicine and requires a fundamentally different view not only of evidence, but of what it means for practice to be based on evidence" (p. 300).

Like Sackett et al. (1996), Rolfe and Gardner (2005) call for a partnership of evidence. They write, "By incorporating EBP into a reflective/reflexive cycle that brings together practice and research, nurses can shift the focus of their care from people to persons and thereby develop a science of the unique that will respond to the needs of the individual" (p. 308).

In sum, hierarchies of evidence continue to limit narrative-based evidence, negatively impacting the full potential of nursing's medicine. It is time for nursing education to expand its understanding of evidence to include the full partnership of quantitative and qualitative data. Like other social structures, the nursing profession must evaluate its own position on the domination/partnership continuum, identifying ways it supports domination so it can then chart paths towards partnership.

Partnership in Nursing Education

In *Tomorrow's Children: A Blueprint for Partnership Education in the 21st Century* (2000), Eisler states there are three interconnected core components in partnership education: process, content, and structure. These components describe *how* we learn and teach, *what* we learn and teach, and *where* we learn and teach. This is a very useful framework for addressing significant challenges in current nursing education.

Process: How We Teach

Nursing faculty can base their pedagogies (teaching philosophies) on principles of partnership or principles of domination. In partnership-based nursing education, professors recognize that each student comes into nursing already possessing a rich set of experiences and knowledge. Each student also has unique learning styles and preferred methods of retention.

Partnership educators do not treat students as blank slates or empty vessels ready to be filled. They acknowledge and develop multiple forms of intelligence—especially emotional intelligence. In partnership-based nursing education, faculty and students cocreate knowledge. Students are encouraged to take an active role in their own knowledge development. Questions are encouraged and transdisciplinary generation of knowledge is promoted.

Partnership-based nursing faculties facilitate, instead of control, learning. They know each student as a unique individual and therefore guide learning according to the student's learning styles and current knowledge level. This allows students to be fully engaged with their own learning. Furthermore, partnership-based nursing education offers students opportunities for self-directed learning as well as opportunities to collaborate. Both skill sets are valued and developed.

The absence of fear is perhaps the most important characteristic of the teacher-student relationship in partnership-based nursing education. Students feel safe knowing that both their insights and questions are respected. Similarly, when students take exams to evaluate their learning, they feel safe knowing the exams test their knowledge of content rather than their ability to figure out a specific teacher's style of writing. In their clinical experiences, students in a partnership relationship with their faculty know they can safely ask questions, make observations they feel indicate patient status changes, and challenge orders or medications that appear to be incorrect. Having the opportunity to learn and apply these skills is critical for safe and effective nursing practice.

PROCESS: HOW WE TEACH

To illustrate the difference between a domination and partnership approach to how we teach, consider the following scenarios. These reflect two different paradigms when orienting students to the norms of the classroom.

continues

continued

Teacher: *Welcome to Nursing 101. I am Dr. Smith, and I will be teaching you what you need to know to be a success. Look to your left and look to your right. By the end of this program, only one of you will remain, only one of you will succeed. Therefore, you need to work harder than you have ever worked in your life, or you won't make it. I am not here to babysit you. You have to do the work. I only want to hear questions after you have thought things through very carefully for yourself. If you do not learn this content well, you can kill people out in clinicals, so my exams are very, very difficult. My job is to protect the public, so I will make sure only the best and brightest students graduate to be nurses.*

This obviously was a domination approach, given the following characteristics:

- *Threats are used to create fear of failure.*

- *There is a hierarchy of domination where the teacher knows everything and the students do not know anything. Communication and learning flow only one direction.*

- *Competition is the norm for the classroom rather than collaboration.*

- *Patronizing language is used, and questions are discouraged.*

- *Focus is placed on the likelihood of failure rather than the likelihood of success, and the teacher's primary role is that of being a gatekeeper.*

Now let's see the same orientation with partnership-based teaching.

Teacher: *Welcome to Nursing 101. I am Dr. Smith, and I will be your faculty for this course. Together we will be shaping a learning community where each of us will bring knowledge and experiences from our past and our clinicals to the classroom. I want our theory content and our practice experiences to be seamlessly connected; therefore, we will be sharing many stories to illustrate the nursing knowledge that is necessary for quality care. Look to your right and look to your left. These are your colleagues, and together you will reach your goal of becoming a nurse. I urge you to form study groups as early as possible because each of you will help each other understand the content over the course of this semester. I am here to walk beside you and help each of you move toward your highest potential. We are partners in learning, therefore, I need to know when something I say is not clear or a concept does not make sense. Chances are if you have a question, others around you also have the same question. So please raise* *your hand and let me know if you need more explanation. You need to take the exams on your own, as they test individual knowledge, but I am very willing to discuss test-taking skills with any of you if you want to see me before an exam. We will also review exams once the scores are posted so you know the best way to prepare for future exams. My goal is to see you succeed.*

The scenario includes the following partnership characteristics:

- *Encouragement creates hope for success.*

- *There is a hierarchy of actualization where the teacher uses power to lift up rather than put down. Communication flows both ways, and students are respected for the knowledge they already possess and are encouraged to bring to the classroom.*

- *Collaboration is promoted as the norm in and out of the classroom.*

- *Questions are encouraged, which directly impacts the nurses' future ability to critically think and be risk-takers.*

- *Emphasis is placed on success rather than failure, and the teacher's primary role is to work with each individual student to help him or her succeed.*

Content: What We Teach

Another way partnership-based nursing education promotes a deeper level of knowledge acquisition is that it recognizes multiple knowledge sources. Partnership faculties teach the entire *BASE of Nursing* (Potter, 2013).

Partnership educators encourage students to develop a deep sense of presence with those they serve, be it individual patients or whole communities. Through that presence, relationships are built and an environment is created where narratives can be revealed. Narratives hold a great amount of data—data that is often missed when only objective and numerical measurements are obtained. Narrative data combined with best practice guidelines allow nurses, patients, and communities to cocreate true healing.

When professors use a partnership-based approach to nursing education, they develop a deep sense of presence with their students and create a relationship based on trust. This trust-based relationship allows faculty to elicit stories about their clinical experiences and reflections about coursework and assignments from their students. They use these valuable narratives to create effective curriculum content. Partnership-based nursing faculty also use narratives to illuminate best practice standards and to demonstrate essential nursing interventions. The entire teaching/learning experience in the partnership paradigm is therefore both reflective and reflexive.

In partnership-based nursing education, hierarchies of evidence do not guide curriculum content. Narratives and relationships are emphasized just as much as quantitative and objective content. This approach supports one of the key recommendations in *Educating Nurses: A Call for Radical Transformation* (Benner, Sutphen, Leonard, & Day, 2010). In this book, the authors state:

> *Learning to think like a nurse involves developing skill with narrative structures and narrative thinking; an understanding of the clinical situation; the ability to find science-based answers to pathophysiology, therapies, signs and symptoms; and the relational and communication skills of listening to and clarifying patient and family concerns. Because injuries and illness occur in the context of a person's life, the nurse must formulate a narrative of the patient's immediate clinical history, his [or her] concerns, and even an account of [her or] his life and lifeworld. (p. 225)*

Nursing care is dependent on partnership-based relationships. Therefore, this is critical content to include in all levels of nursing education.

Nursing history content, as you read in Chapter 4, is another critical element in partnership-based nursing education. Curriculum should help students make the connection between the devaluation of nursing (a profession mainly composed of women) and the cultural devaluation we have inherited of women and anything stereotypically associated with women or the "feminine." Nurses need to understand that much that is taught as knowledge and truth in the educational canon reflects this devaluation and how this limits ways of knowing and being that challenge systems of domination.

CONTENT: WHAT WE TEACH

Curriculum A (reinforcing domination-based content): Recent emphasis on evidence-based practice is finally earning the nursing profession the recognition it deserves. Other professions can now trust nurses to be qualified partners in patient care. In the past nurses were considered the "handmaidens" of physicians, but this is no longer the case. Today's nurses use critical thinking to apply best practice interventions for their patients.

Curriculum B (encouraging partnership-based nursing): Throughout nursing history, nursing leaders have put themselves in a place where they could listen with empathy to the experiences of the individuals and communities they serve. From that deep listening, stories emerged. They then used the stories to create new and innovative models of care, ranging from public health and school nursing to education programs for community midwives. These visionary leaders combined the knowledge and strengths of the people they served with the best practice knowledge of the time, resulting in quantifiable health care outcomes and improved patient and community satisfaction.

We will have more to say about content in partnership education in subsequent chapters. But here we briefly want to move on to the third, interconnected, element of partnership education: partnership structure.

Structure: Where We Teach

As we move into partnership-based nursing education, we want to create environments where rigid professional hierarchies are challenged. This requires flexibility in designing practicum sites to ensure they include intentional experiences of interprofessional practice. We also want to create structures where our students' understanding of the spheres of nursing is expanded, in other words, structures that support the teaching of partnership content and provide an opportunity to experience partnership roles.

Traditionally, nursing clinical education has focused primarily on acute care, with limited experience of public health or community care. This model of practice needs to be restructured to emphasize community-based partnerships. For example, students can observe community health workers to see their roles. They can provide services in school-based clinics for adolescents. They can follow community faith nurses as they round on families who attend their synagogues, mosques, or churches. Reenvisioning where we teach allows nurse educators to use the best partnership for their students.

A partnership structure also models what Eisler (2002) calls *hierarchies of actualization* rather than hierarchies of domination. In actualization hierarchies, respect and accountability flow both ways, rather than from the bottom up only, as in hierarchies of domination. Hierarchies of actualization facilitate the empowerment of students and often are essential to counter the socialization of women (who still are the majority of nurses) to devalue themselves. All this is, of course, also important for men, since men who embrace nursing still have to contend with socialization that the male gender is not qualified to provide nurture and care.

In summarizing *Tomorrow's Children* (2000) Eisler writes, "I want to invite not only parents, students, primary- and secondary-school teachers, university professors, and other educators, but also all those working for a better future, to become active partners in developing Partnership Education" (Center for Partnership Studies, n.d.). Now is the time, and here is our invitation, to co-create partnership education in nursing.

STRUCTURE: WHERE WE TEACH

Potter coordinates the Doctor of Nursing Practice in Health Innovation and Leadership (HIL) at the University of Minnesota (U of M). On the first day of class she takes new HIL students on a field trip to the U of M's Medical Device Innovation Center. The students have an opportunity to see innovation labs with cutting-edge technology, including 3-D printers, imaging equipment, and media that allows virtual tours of the heart and other organs. This experience helps move students beyond the siloed thinking of their own discipline and instills core partnership values, including:

- *All knowledge is nursing knowledge.*
- *Nursing knowledge is pertinent to all other fields of study.*

- *Innovation occurs in the interprofessional space between disciplines.*
- *All leadership and innovation experiences, even those outside of nursing, are important for educating transformational nursing leaders.*
- *Nurses hold critical knowledge about patients and health and healing that is required to drive effective health care technology and policy development for the future.*

Partnership Exemplar: An Assignment Designed to Illuminate the Domination/Partnership Continuum

The messages are so ubiquitous, and sometimes so subtle, that most people do not even realize they have been socialized to accept the domination perspective. This socialization begins so early that domination may be the only paradigm some people have ever known. Therefore, nursing faculty must design curriculum content to help students realize there is an alternative and shift from domination to partnership.

Partnership content based on Riane Eisler's cultural transformation theory is woven through the curriculum of the Health Innovation and Leadership Doctor of Nursing Practice (DNP) specialty at the University of Minnesota. For example, Potter (2012b) designed the following assignment to help students see threads of domination and partnership in their personal lives, their work, and society at large. Students were taught elements of the partnership and domination paradigms. Then they were given the whole semester to complete the following assignment.

Journal Assignment

Throughout the semester, observe and collect examples of partnership and domination in our society. These examples can be from lived experiences in the community, television shows, radio, music, newspapers, experiences at your work, experiences at the university, and so on. This does not have to be a formal APA paper, but I do want the source and date (if it is an experience or observation, the date is sufficient) and a brief description of your insights. The final submission can be as informal as bullet points with dates and examples. I will be grading on involvement, depth, and degree of observation (Potter, 2012b).

Selected Student Observations

- **EXAMPLE OF DOMINATION:** "Jon Stewart interviews Steven Brill, author of 'Bitter Pill: Why Medical Bills are Killing US'" (Retrieved from http://beforeitsnews.com/economy/2013/03/jon-stewart-interviews-steven-brill-author-of-bitter-pill-why-medical-bills-are-killing-us-2496016.html)

  The Brill article shows the domination of the hospital charge system that results in exorbitantly inflated billing of patients. The article illustrates the domination of an excessive profit motive in health care and the large profits many hospitals enjoy, thanks to what some might call fraudulent charges to vulnerable patients.

- **EXAMPLE OF PARTNERSHIP:** I was riding the metro: I remember I was daydreaming and realized we were at my stop! I jumped up and said quietly, "Please hold the door!" This message was relayed as "hold the door!" and then louder, "HOLD THE DOOR!!!" and finally someone by the door said, "I'M HOLDING THE DOOR!!!" At this point, everyone is starting to laugh!

  As I'm shuffling through the crowd, because I also had a suitcase I was trying to maneuver through people, I think I heard the bell that the door was going to close. So I said, "Wait! This is my stop!" and again, in echo fashion, I heard, "This is her stop!"; then a few people down, "THIS IS HER STOP"; and finally, "THIS IS HER STOP!!!" More laughter ensued!

  I just made it outside the train and just as the doors were closing behind me, I said, "I love Minnesota!", and true to form, I heard, "She loves

Minnesota"; and it travelled through the train: "She loves Minnesota!" and finally, "SHE LOVES MINNESOTA!" At that time, the train had started moving away, but I remember smiling, and everyone on the metro was laughing and clapping.

I remember feeling very well taken care of by an entire community at that time. It may have been nothing more than "manners" or "Minnesota nice," but it appeared to be a group effort to ensure I made it off at my stop!

- **EXAMPLE OF PARTNERSHIP:** I want to trust myself. I want to partner with myself to reach my full potential. I also want to be more trusting of others and believe that people are innately good and motivated. I want to embrace negotiations as an opportunity for discussion and growth…. Not as moments that have a "winner" and "loser."

- **EXAMPLE OF DOMINATION:** Plumer, B. (2013). America's staggering defense budget, in charts. *The Washington Post*. (Retrieved from http://www.washingtonpost.com/blogs/wonkblog/wp/2013/01/07/everything-chuck-hagel-needs-to-know-about-the-defense-budget-in-charts.)

-The United States spent more than the next 13 nations on national defense in 2011.

-I know that defense needs to be a portion of our nation's budget, but when I see these numbers, it seems our nation clearly prioritizes domination over partnership.

-I wonder what numbers would look like if we added up costs of partnership endeavors and compared these costs to defense costs.

-It would be an interesting discussion of the culture of our nation and where citizens feel we should go from here.

- **EXAMPLE OF PARTNERSHIP** (Boston, April 15, 2013)

On Monday, April 15, 2013, explosives were planted at the Boston Marathon, an important day in the community that always occurs on the holiday Patriots' Day.

In the days following the bombing more and more stories of partnership emerged:

- Hospitals from nearby states sent food for staff and flew in blood as needed.

- Orthopedic residents could not call the hospitals or each other because phone lines were down. They jumped on their email list serve…sending appropriate numbers to all the facilities.

- Community members gave blood, and employees of the blood bank worked round the clock to replenish stores.

- The Boston community rallied: Individuals were kind, really kind. Saying "thank you" and "I love you" to each other so frequently I wondered where I had teleported to.

- Sometimes in the darkest moments, there is the most partnership.

- **EXAMPLE OF DOMINATION:** During a meeting with a group of DNP (Doctor of Nursing Practice) graduates, a new topic came to light that was an example of the domination culture established by physicians at my hospital:

  - One of the DNP graduates is a nurse practitioner who recently requested more business cards be made. On her new set of business cards the organization refused to allow her to have DNP listed. When she inquired about the reason, she was told that the title DNP is not required in order to be a nurse practitioner, and thus it could not be included. However, physicians at the institution have MD, PhD or MD, MBA frequently listed on their cards. Their PhD and MBA degrees are not "required" for their position as physicians at the hospital, but they are allowed to list their degrees.

This is an example of how physicians have worked to suppress nurses at the organization. Physicians at the organization have frequently complained that the DNP degree makes the roles of nurses too confusing. What was their solution? Do not allow nurses to take credit for their doctoral education.

- **EXAMPLE OF PARTNERSHIP:** I will admit that this semester has been a time of intense and deep change for me. My eyes and heart are open to dynamics around me that I was not aware of before. I have new words and learning to better define how I feel and perceive within myself, and the world around me...I now can better understand the concept that indeed we are imperfect and broken beings who inhabit an imperfect and broken world, and our calling is to use our human capacity to direct these tensions in a positive way to generate insight, energy, and new life.

- **EXAMPLE OF DOMINATION:** One of our assignments in [another DNP nursing course] was a group writing assignment regarding engaging patients in shared decision-making in the context of evidence-based practice.

  - In reading the other assignment offerings from other teams, I was disappointed. I will remind you that all the groups are nurses working on advanced practice degrees. Many of the groups rejected shared decision-making because they stated that patients did not really want it, and they supported their thoughts with evidence!

  - Many of them talked about shared decision-making as a necessary evil, a hoop that had to be jumped through to get patients to do what they wanted them to do.

  - One group even used the word comply. Some of the synonyms for comply are obey, consent, and conform, which do not bring the thought of partnership to mind. There is much to do to lead nursing back to partnership so that nursing can then lead their patients back to partnership.

- **EXAMPLE OF PARTNERSHIP:** Our current health care system has for years excluded patients from being active participants in their care, favored disease management over health management, and taught our patients that providers, and not they, will be the sole decision-makers of care delivery. We should then not be surprised when our patients expect us to care for them and provide treatments on demand, and are displeased when we do not make good on our assumed promise that we will care for them, and that their participation is not required nor welcome.

It will take much undoing to reengage our patients in their own health and health care when we have a system that has not fostered these behaviors. However, we CAN do it, and understanding our patients is our first diagnostic step in the journey.

- **EXAMPLE OF PARTNERSHIP:** As I continue to consider and work on my DNP project, I continue to read and learn. I ordered all of Riane Eisler's books, and they travel with me so I can read in the few moments I have during my travel days. I find her teachings comforting and hopeful and aligned to my nursing vision of the future.

Conclusion

These reflections demonstrate that the assignment helped the students begin seeing aspects of domination and partnership in the world around them. We know from the *nursing process* (assess, diagnose, plan, implement, evaluate) that you cannot effectively apply a nursing intervention until you have carefully assessed and diagnosed the problem. Similarly, nurses cannot hope to be effective agents of change, supporting and manifesting characteristics of partnership, until they can recognize and challenge threads of domination. Being able to recognize patterns of domination and partnership is a core competency in partnership-based nursing education. Nursing faculty, we are calling on you to lead the way.

PRINCIPLES OF PARTNERSHIP-BASED NURSING EDUCATION

- *Rather than starting with a blank slate, learning begins with each student's unique life experiences, skills, and knowledge.*

- *Students are seen as partners in the learning process. The student is an expert in her or his own knowledge and experience. The role of the instructor, therefore, is to create hierarchies of actualization. In hierarchies of actualization, teachers use power with students rather than over students (Eisler, 2002) to cocreate learning.*

- *Faculty inspires and models facilitation rather than control.*

- *Each student's unique abilities are fostered.*
- *Diverse learning styles are honored.*
- *Students' voices are heard, and their ideas are respected.*
- *Emotional needs are understood and addressed.*
- *Cooperative learning and individual responsibility are combined.*
- *Learning is a reciprocal activity between teacher and student.*
- *Students learn through experiential opportunities, and these opportunities can be cocreated.*
- *Students think for themselves and trust their observations and experiences.*
- *Rigid hierarchies are strongly discouraged. Students learn to value both the shared and unique contributions of all the professions.*
- *Students are helped to identify patterns of domination and partnership in health care and society at large.*
- *Nursing history reflects the essential role nurses have played and continue to play.*
- *Students are taught to use the lenses of the domination and partnership model in their studies, work, and lives.*
- *Students are made aware of the hidden subtext of gendered values that has disempowered nurses and led to dysfunctional policies and practices in health care.*
- *Narratives and relationships are emphasized just as much as quantitative and objective content.*
- *Students are encouraged to engage patients as partners and to pay close attention to patients' perspectives and narratives.*
- *Students are encouraged to question, and their voices are heard.*
- *Students are encouraged to be partnership leaders.*

Adapted from Riane Eisler's (2000) book Tomorrow's Children: A Blueprint for Partnership Education in the 21st Century.

References

Benner, P. (1984). *From novice to expert: Excellence and power in clinical nursing practice*. Menlo Park, CA: Addison-Wesley Publishing Company.

Benner, P. (2012). Urgently needed: A radical transformation of professional collaboration and teamwork. Retrieved from http://www.educatingnurses.com/articles/interprofessional-education/

Benner, P., Sutphen, M., Leonard, V., & Day, L. (2010). *Educating nurses: A call for radical transformation*. San Francisco, CA: Jossey-Bass.

Center for Partnership Studies. (n.d.). Excerpt from the prologue to *Tomorrow's Children*. Retrieved from http://www.partnershipway.org/learn-more/other-books-incorporating-partnership/preview/excerpt-from-the-foreword-of-tomorrows-children

Claridge, J. A., & Fabian, T. C. (2005). History and development of evidence-based medicine. *World Journal of Surgery, 29*(5), 547-553.

Cochrane Collaboration. (n.d.a). Archie Cochrane: The name behind the Cochrane collaboration. Retrieved from http://www.cochrane.org/about-us/history/archie-cochrane

Cochrane Collaboration. (n.d.b). Evidence-based health care. Retrieved from http://www.cochrane.org/about-us/evidence-based-health-care

Cochrane Collaboration. (n.d.c). About us. Retrieved from http://www.cochrane.org/about-us

Eisler, R. (2000). *Tomorrow's children: A blueprint for partnership education in the 21st century*. Boulder, CO: Westview Press.

Eisler, R. (2002). *The power of partnership: Seven relationships that will change your life*. Novato, CA: New World Library.

Frenk, J., Chen, L., Bhutta, Z. A., Cohen, J., Crisp, N., Evans, T.,...Zurayk, H. (November, 2010). Health professionals for a new century: Transforming education to strengthen health systems in an interdependent world. *The Lancet, 376*(9756), 1923-1958.

Greenhalgh, T. (1997). How to read a paper: Getting your bearings (deciding what the paper is about). *BMJ: British Medical Journal, 315*, 243-246.

Greenhalgh, T. (1999). Narrative based medicine: Narrative based medicine in an evidence based world. *BMJ: British Medical Journal, 318*, 323-325.

Institute of Medicine. (2010). *The future of nursing: Leading change, advancing health*. Washington, DC: National Academies Press.

International Council of Nurses (ICN). (2010). *Definition of nursing*. Retrieved from http://www.icn.ch/about-icn/icn-definition-of-nursing/

Potter, T. (2012a). Educating for partnering. *Creative Nursing, 18*(2), 47-49.

Potter, T. (2012b). *NURS7606: Relationship-based leadership*. Unpublished syllabus, School of Nursing, University of Minnesota, United States.

Potter, T. M. (2013). *The BASE of nursing*. Unpublished manuscript, School of Nursing, University of Minnesota, United States of America.

Randle, J. (2003). Changes in self-esteem during a 3-year pre-registration Diploma in Higher Education (Nursing) programme. *Journal of Clinical Nursing, 12*(1), 142-143.

Robert Wood Johnson Foundation. (2012). Enduring trust: Nurses again top Gallup's poll on honesty and ethics. Retrieved from http://www.rwjf.org/en/blogs/human-capital-blog/2012/12/enduring_trust_nurs.html

Rolfe, G., & Gardner, L. (2005). Towards a nursing science of the unique: Evidence, reflexivity and the study of persons. *Journal of Research in Nursing, 10*(3), 297-310.

Sackett, D. L., Rosenberg, W. M. C., Muir Gray, J. A., Haynes, B., & Richardson, W. S. (1996). Evidence based medicine: What it is and what it isn't: It's about integrating individual clinical expertise and the best external evidence. *BMJ: British Medical Journal, 312*(7023), 71-72.

World Health Organization (WHO). (2011). *World health statistics 2011*. Geneva, Switzerland: WHO Press.

Chapter 7

Self-Care, Professional Identity, and Self-Efficacy: The Foundations of Caring

"Never be bullied into silence. Never allow yourself to be made a victim. Accept no one's definition of your life, but define yourself."
—Attributed to Harvey Fierstein

You know the drill: The plane has just taken off and the flight attendant with a bored smile reviews the safety instructions. "Should the plane lose pressure, oxygen masks will drop from the ceiling. Please secure your own mask first before helping others." They have to tell people that because many people are wired to help others first, especially in an emergency. This basic safety message also applies to nursing: To be safe, make sure you take care of yourself. Otherwise, you will not be any use to others, and you may even cause harm.

One reason self-care is so critical in nursing is because stress and its related *compassion fatigue* are major precursors to nurses leaving the profession prematurely. With the current and projected severe nursing shortage (Americans for Nursing Shortage Relief Alliance, 2012; Buerhaus, Auerbach, & Staiger, 2009), anything that threatens the well-being of nurses must be addressed. The biggest stressors not only for nurses, but also for other health care professionals, are the persistent patterns of domination in our current health care system.

Identifying Patterns of Domination

Nursing has always been a stressful profession. But recently more and more complaints of adverse levels of stress are coming forward. Jennings (2008) suggests that the escalating stress experienced by nurses might be directly related to the increasing demands of technology, rising health care costs, resource shortages, and dysfunctional work environment communication. In the article "Transforming Health Care: A Safety Imperative," national quality and safety experts write:

> *Many physicians do not know how to be team players and regard other health workers as assistants. Outmoded hierarchical structures inhibit collaboration and learning. Nurses are trapped in rigid organizational structures in which they often spend more time tending to their records than to their patients. Often, their work environment does not permit them to realize their full potential. (Leape et al., 2009, p. 424-425)*

This article identifies some patterns of domination that will now be discussed in more detail.

Technology: Electronic Medical Records

The world is in the midst of a technological revolution so transformative that we may not fully grasp what happened until we emerge on the other side. Consider for a moment the two previous technological revolutions experienced by humanity: the agricultural revolution and the industrial revolution. Both of these major technological shifts radically transformed the way humans interact with one another and their natural environment. These earlier technological revolutions impacted every institution, including family, education, economics, government, and even religion. You can imagine that previous to and during both revolutions, when things started to shift, there was doubt, fear, resistance, and various levels of willingness to make the change.

The digital revolution we are currently undergoing is no less dramatic or significant than the previous revolutions. The digital revolution began in the latter part of the 20th century with the arrival of the personal computer and cell phone. Similar to the upheaval caused by the previous revolutions, the digital revolution is eliciting a spectrum of emotions ranging from doubt and fear to various levels of engagement with the change.

One of the most significant changes in health care related to the digital revolution is the arrival of the *electronic medical record (EMR;* Institute of Medicine [IOM], 2003). An EMR is a legal clinical record that is created with a computer and stored digitally. EMRs document specific health care events such as a clinic visit or a hospitalization. Key features of the EMR include a clinical data repository, a clinical decision support system, a controlled medical vocabulary, a computerized order entry system, and related documentation applications (Garets & Davis, 2005).

When EMRs eventually become the standard, widespread use of electronic health records (EHRs) will become the norm. EHRs are summaries of care provided to individual clients by multiple care delivery organizations (CDOs) within an integrated system. The use of EHRs will allow health care consumers and providers to have access to longitudinal health records or summaries of health care provided over time (Garets & Davis, 2005)—a matter discussed more fully later in this chapter.

One of the chief benefits of these kinds of records is the reduction of costly redundancies (Menachemi & Collum, 2011). When all health care providers have access to the same client health records, they can see what has been ordered before and thereby base their clinical decisions on complete data. Having all the data in one place is especially important in cases where patients have one or more chronic illnesses. For example, it is not uncommon for clients living with chronic illnesses to have numerous health care providers, including a primary provider and one or more specialists. Without a shared record, providers might repeat costly diagnostic tests and double-prescribe medications and treatments. This problem is compounded when patients frequently change providers or provide inaccurate or incomplete patient histories.

Another potential use of EMRs and EHRs is that providers and researchers will be able to *mine* or extract important data from these records to predict at-risk populations and provide early, cost-effective treatment plans. For example, mining data from large volumes of patient EMRs and EHRs may reveal patterns that we cannot see when we care for individuals (Jaret, 2013). We may, for instance, learn that patients taking certain combinations of medications have more incidents of falls. Having this information would allow nurses to do interventions to decrease the risk of falls. Nurses can then also teach families how to prevent falls when a patient is being discharged home.

This backstory illustrates some of the benefits of EMRs. However, EMRs present quandaries by creating new or additional nursing role expectations.

Until recently, most of an acute care nurse's time was spent in direct provision of care or patient/family education. Unit nurses may have called a physician or nurse practitioner or done summary charting at the end of the shift, but generally time spent at the nurses' station was an exception. With the arrival of EMRs, the allocation of nurses' time has been reprioritized. Now a much larger percentage of time is spent entering data into the computer. Even though in some facilities this may be done bedside via a computer on wheels, charting is a very different way of relating to patients.

Proponents argue EMRs have many timesaving and cost-saving benefits. Critics are concerned that, in addition to taking away from time nurses spend with patients, EMR templates and check boxes fail to capture the rich narrative data essential for patient care decisions (Furst et al., 2013).

When you compare the new role of nurses, prompted by technology, with the BASE of Nursing (Potter, 2013), you can see that being present and stories or narrative-based practice are increasingly marginalized—even though these are the domains that set the medicine of nursing apart from the medicine of physicians. When nurses do not have time to practice their unique medicine, satisfaction with the profession decreases; attrition risk increases.

A partnership approach to technology would involve several changes related to EMRs. First of all, rather than EMRs, all electronic charting would be included under EHRs, so everyone is clear that the records are shared equally by the entire team: patients, nurses, physicians, therapists, and other health care team members. Furthermore, when nurses work in a partnership-oriented system, they can codesign or have input into any technological change that impacts their work. For instance, they get to help design the content of the EHRs so they reflect the full range of care that nurses provide. In addition to content, nurses can also codesign the EHR process. They partner with information technology (IT) to give input so that data fields can be quickly and efficiently accessed and thereby free their time for meaningful caring such as being present and listening to patient narratives.

ELECTRONIC HEALTH RECORDS: BENEFITS AND CHALLENGES

Benefits:

- *Decreased duplication of diagnostic tests*

- *Decreased risk of medication errors*

- *Presents information in a way that is accessible to the entire team*

- *Supports interprofessional collaboration*

- *Can remain with the health care consumer their entire lifetime, no matter where or how many times they relocate*

- *May eventually be used to identify potential health care risks and educate the health care consumer on important health care decisions*

- *The electronic health record also holds the potential to make previously invisible and nonbillable nursing care more visible. It is hoped respect for nurses will increase with increased use of EHR.*

continues

continued

Challenges:

- *The record is only as good as the required content fields. Potentially they can miss significant data, especially narrative data.*

- *Individuals who do not understand the lived experience of health care workers may design the record. Therefore, internal logic may be missing.*

- *The process of completing the record may take time away from relationships with patients.*

- *Even when computers are in the patient rooms, the provider may lack the ability to be present to both the patient or family and the record at the same time.*

- *The two-dimensional and visual nature of the EHR may decrease the health care provider's sensory acuity and ability to pick up subtle data from other senses.*

Rising Health Care Costs

The rising costs of health care continue to impact nursing in negative ways, causing increasing stress to both nurses and patients. Before President Obama signed the Patient Protection and Affordable Care Act (PPACA) into law, uninsured or underinsured patients often waited until their condition was critical before seeking health care. Most people will not use preventive measures or simple and effective early treatments if they have to pay for the full cost of services out of their own pocket. This failure to seek timely care can cause despair to nurses, who know that doing simple interventions early can prevent suffering and the need for high-cost services later.

Nurses are also being negatively impacted by the implementation of some of the initiatives to contain health care costs, especially for Medicare and Medicaid patients. One of the initiatives is the Hospital Consumer Assessment of Healthcare Providers and Systems (HCAHPS), the first national standardized, publicly reported survey documenting patients' hospitalization experiences. The HCAHPS scores measure the following:

- How well nurses and doctors communicate with patients

- How responsive hospital staff are to patients' needs

- How well hospital staff help patients manage pain

- How well the staff communicates with patients about medicines

- Whether key information is provided at discharge (Centers for Medicare and Medicaid Services, 2012)

In principle these are sensible measures. However, as a part of the 2005 Deficit Reduction Act, hospitals must submit their aggregated HCAHPS scores to receive their full annual payment for care of Medicare and Medicaid patients. Because these scores are primarily related to nursing care or nursing supervision of other team members, the responsibility for attaining high scores falls primarily to the nurses. And if staffing is poor or there is lack of administrator support, this can be an impossible task for nurses.

If nurses do not feel they have the power to intervene in effective ways, they feel the sense of powerlessness and hopelessness that has been called *moral distress* (Edward & Hercelinskyj, 2007; Pendry, 2007; Zuzelo, 2007). Moral distress is defined as "a phenomenon in which one knows the right action to take, but is constrained from taking it" (Epstein & Delgado, 2010). The adverse impact of this on nurses has been well documented.

Corley (2002) found 26% of nurses' resignations were related to moral distress. Findings of Manojlovich's (2005b) survey of 376 bedside nurses also indicate that moral distress and low self-efficacy strongly correlate with job dissatisfaction. She wrote:

Not believing in their ability to mobilize the necessary motivation, cognitive resources, and courses of action necessary to control their work, nurses may choose to stay out of patients' rooms and disengage themselves from intense healthcare situations. They may choose to spend time at the nurses' station with each other, rather than with patients, walking to patients' rooms only when assigned tasks must be carried out. While dysfunctional from a professional practice viewpoint, this behavior serves the purpose of reducing stress in an otherwise intolerable situation. (pp. 276-277)

The women and anger study conducted by Droppleman and Thomas (1996) includes a database of 500 interviews with women from different professions. The authors concluded that much of the anger, frustration, and exhaustion experienced by nurse participants was directly related to their perceived inability to effect change. In addition, the researchers also found that feelings of powerlessness were cited as a major cause of job dissatisfaction. Droppleman and Thomas (1996) suggested that perceived powerlessness in nurses was related to numerous factors, including the socialization of women and the lack of information about the development and use of power. For example, nurses may learn to think negatively about power when they experience abusive forms of power so common in the domination paradigm. Nurses need to learn that they have a choice and can follow principles of partnership, using power to promote quality and safety for their patients.

On a positive note, high HCAHPS scores and consequently higher rates of reimbursement for the health care system are directly tied to the care provided by nurses. Under these circumstances, nurses can demonstrate the value of their care in a way that is tangible for those who direct the business of health care.

It is not difficult to see that a partnership approach to nursing care is likely to correlate with higher HCHPS scores. Among other results, partnership improves interprofessional communication, promotes patient-centered care, and empowers patients by treating them as partners in their own health via thorough teaching.

Dysfunctional Communication in the Work Environment

Chapter 9 explores the topic of dysfunctional communications in more depth, discussing the relationships between nurses and other nurses. Chapter 10 discusses interprofessional practice. This chapter focuses on the stress many nurses experience due to their work environment and the role communication plays.

Of course, some stressful conditions are inevitable aspects of health care—for example, the death of patients—but other conditions can be altered (Coeling & Cukr, 2000; Manojlovich, 2005a). One such condition, which is a major cause of stress for nurses in their workplaces, is verbal abuse from other professionals. Manderino and Berkey (1997) surveyed 130 staff nurses with a Verbal Abuse Questionnaire and found that over 90% of respondents had experienced verbal abuse at least once within the past year, while the average number of reported abuse events was 6–12 times a year. The authors reported that the most damaging forms of abuse were abusive anger, ignoring, and condescension.

In 2002, Rosenstein surveyed 1,200 nurses, physicians, and hospital executives to examine how disruptive physician behavior impacts nurse satisfaction, morale, and retention. When asked if they had personally witnessed or experienced disruptive behaviors, 92.5% of the respondents said they had. The disruptive behaviors cited most frequently included yelling, condescension, disrespect, berating patients, berating colleagues, and using inappropriate language. Disruptive behaviors on average were reported to happen one to two times a month.

According to Rosenstein's 2002 study, nurses reported that these disruptive behaviors were most likely to happen in the following situations:

- After placing calls to physicians
- After questioning or seeking to clarify physicians' orders
- When physicians thought their orders were not being carried out correctly or in a timely manner
- After perceived delays in delivery of care
- After sudden changes in patient status (p. 32)

Many of these nursing actions are directly related to safe patient care. Therefore, behaviors that make nurses hesitant to question unsafe orders or afraid to call regarding patient status changes not only compromise the quality of patient care but can lead to worsening conditions and possible death (Page, 2004).

The Institute for Safe Medication Practices (Brehio, 2004) in a survey of 2,000 health professionals found that 7% of the respondents were involved in a medication error in which intimidation was a contributing factor, and 49% reported that experiences with intimidation impact the way they question or clarify medical orders. Findings showed:

> At least once in the past year, about 40% of all respondents who had concerns about the safety of a medication error assumed that it was correct rather than interact with an intimidating prescriber. Even when the prescriber was questioned about safety, almost half (49%) of respondents felt pressured into dispensing a product or administering a medication despite their concerns. (p. 1)

Based on these results, the Institute for Safe Medications Practices (Brehio, 2004) made recommendations that, if implemented, would move health care systems closer to a partnership model for interprofessional relationships. These recommendations include zero tolerance of intimidation, increasing the value placed on team cohesion, according the highest value to patient protection, and preventing poor behavior related to hierarchies of domination.

You might be tempted to think that by now our culture must have moved beyond the domination behaviors experienced by nurses described in these studies. However, in her *New York Times* article "Physician, Heel Thyself," Brown (2011) reports:

> It was morning rounds in the hospital and the entire medical team stood in the patient's room. A test result was late, and the patient, a friendly, middle-aged man, jokingly asked his doctor whom he should yell at. Turning and pointing at the patient's nurse, the doctor replied, "If you want to scream at anyone, scream at her." This vignette is not a scene from the medical drama "House," nor did it take place 30 years ago, when nurses were considered

subservient to doctors. Rather, it happened just a few months ago, at my hospital, to me. As we walked out of the patient's room I asked the doctor if I could quote him in an article. "Sure," he answered. "It's a time-honored tradition, blame the nurse whenever anything goes wrong." These adverse behaviors toward nurses are not inevitable. They are directly related to health care systems that allow domination behaviors to continue without being challenged. (The Opinion Pages)

Powerlessness

Nurses' perception that they are powerless is a common theme in many studies. Literature indicates that nurses experience powerlessness in the face of technology that negatively impacts time with their patients; powerlessness in the face of increasing expectations yet limited health care resources; and powerlessness related to dysfunctional communication with dominating physicians (Attridge, 1996). Manojlovich (2007) summarizes these factors as the degree to which nurses have control over the content of nursing practice, the context of nursing practice, and competence related to nursing practice. In other words, when the professional identity of nurses is defined and managed by non-nurses, a sense of powerlessness prevails.

The perception by nurses that they are powerless and the factors that lead to this perception have profound implications for the ability of nurses to participate as full partners in the redesign of health care in America (IOM, 2010). Journalists Buresh and Gordon (2000) provide an example of one of these factors. When they examined sources for news coverage about health issues, they found that while physicians were quoted more significantly than any other occupational group, nurses were quoted so rarely that they trailed all other professions. Buresh and Gordon concluded, "If there was little trace of nursing in the serious coverage of health and health care, then how could anyone, including those in a position to supply nursing with needed resources, understand and recognize its value" (p. 3).

Accordingly, Buresh and Gordon (2000) report the following examples of nurses' unwillingness to make their voices heard:

- "Nurses, many reporters tell us, seem terrified of expressing strong opinions and seem overly concerned they might offend someone" (p. 4).

- "There is a profound ambivalence in nursing about whether it is even advisable to be more visible, more vocal" (p. 5).

- "Underlying their arguments, however, is a real fear that increasing the 'voice' and 'visibility' of nurses and nursing will bring harm" (p. 34).

The preceding points are further evidence of the urgent need for a partnership model of health care that ensures that the full value of nurses—including the value of their voices—is recognized by other care providers, the media, and nurses themselves.

Partnership With Ourselves

The degree to which we are able to relate to ourselves in a healthy way correlates with our ability to partner with others. This is especially true in health care, where therapeutic communication is essential. The ability to be a partner with ourselves depends on many ingredients, especially strong self-efficacy and a partnership-based work environment.

Self-Efficacy

For nurses to be full partners in interprofessional teams requires that nurses themselves no longer feel powerless. Indeed, Laschinger, Finegan, and Shamian (2001) suggest that patient satisfaction and care outcomes may ultimately be tied to the empowerment and self-efficacy of nurses. Therefore, nurses need to develop strong self-efficacy. Manojlovich (2005b) describes *self-efficacy* as "belief in one's capabilities to organize and execute the courses of action needed to produce the given results" (p. 271). Thus, self-efficacy includes a clear sense of self-identity, control over ways of knowing, and control over ways of relating.

Empowered nurses fully manifest the BASE of Nursing (Potter, 2013), thereby ensuring the most favorable patient care outcomes. As Manojlovich (2007) writes, "Only the bedside nurse, who is in closest proximity to the patient, can fully appreciate subtle patient cues and trends as they arise and act on them to properly care for that patient" ("Control Over the Content of Nursing Practice" section). When nurses have a high degree of self-efficacy, it becomes possible for them to reach their full professional potential.

Self-efficacy is the product of many factors. Nursing education can be a major contributor to a belief in one's capacities. However, there are other factors—especially the degree to which the nursing environment orients to the partnership or the domination model.

Partnership and Empowerment

The social organization of systems (for example, health care) has a major impact on whether nurses do or do not feel empowered. Kanter's theory of social empowerment (as cited in Manojlovich, 2007) states that empowerment is directly tied to whether all employees across all levels of an organization have opportunities and shared power. According to Kanter, employee self-efficacy has less to do with the personality of individuals and more to do with social organization itself. Similarly, Kanter (as cited in Laschinger, Finegan, & Shamian, 2001) notes that access to information and resources, supportive relationships, and the opportunity to learn and grow significantly impact empowerment.

Based on Kanter's theory, health care organizations that operate according to partnership principles can have a powerful impact on the self-efficacy of individual employees. In partnership systems, power is not used *as power over* employees, but to *empower* employees. As much as possible, power is shared, gender balance promotes opportunities, teamwork and relationship-based practice is encouraged, and innovation and creativity are valued (Eisler & Montuori, 2001). All of these partnership principles contribute to a work environment that supports self-efficacy and increased employee satisfaction.

These environments also promote psychological empowerment, which in turn leads to a sense of self-efficacy. Organizations that orient toward the partnership model implement structures that empower employees to positively respond to external factors, including the use of technology, the cost of health care and resource allocation, and rapidly evolving health care policies.

Psychological empowerment consists of four domains: meaning, competence, choice, and impact (Spreitzer, 1995). Wang and Lee (2009) synthesize the literature about these domains as follows:

- *Meaning* "refers to the value of a task goal or purpose, judged in relation to an individual's own ideals or standards. It reflects intrinsic interest in a task and involves a fit between work role requirements and one's beliefs and values" (p. 273).

- *Competence* "is the degree to which an employee feels he or she is able to perform tasks with skill" (p. 273).

- *Choice* "is the sense of autonomy in initiating and regulating work and reflects the degree of self-determination in work behaviors and processes.... Choice is a key component of intrinsic motivation, leading to learning, interest, and resilience in the face of adversity" (p. 273).

- *Impact* is the degree to which individuals feel that they can "influence strategic, administrative, or operating outcomes at work.... Impact is associated with high performance and an absence of withdrawal from difficult situations" (p. 273).

The Center for Partnership Studies (n.d.) lists organizational benefits of partnership systems: Employees feel valued and empowered to participate; they feel safe and less fearful of making mistakes; communication is healthy and open; and employees feel a synergistic sense of community.

EMPOWERING PROFESSIONAL SELF-IDENTITY: A NURSING MANIFESTO

The following statements are from the Nurse Manifest project, an online resource to promote professional self-identity:

"As nurses, we reach for meaningful expressions of our values, too often finding overwhelming constraint and resistance, sometimes within ourselves and

sometimes imposed from without. We are calling for a movement to awaken those precious and powerful ideals that are rooted in nursing's worldwide historical traditions. We believe there are profound possibilities in claiming our individual and professional sovereignty.

"The situation we find ourselves in has been created from an array of forces. While economic issues have helped create a situation in which nurses cannot practice nursing, we, as nurses, have participated by remaining silent. Our professional sovereignty is threatened. The health of global humankind is at risk. It is now time to ask ourselves, who benefits from the situation as it now exists? As long as we know that the current situation inhibits the fullest expression of nursing's highest values, and that people who need our care are not receiving the best we can offer, we know that we, and those we serve, are not benefiting. If nurses are to significantly contribute to a mission of caring for people and communities, we must find our voice, acting now to create situations in which our values come to the center and from which we can realize our best intentions.

"Now, seeking meaningful avenues for action, we choose to identify ourselves with the heritage and future of nurses. From nursing history we have learned the fullness of our own potential as nurses, the strength of nurses, the effect of nurses in communities and to individuals. We have seen our own common self-interest, and common oppression. Having found these authentic bonds as nurses, we realize we can rely on each other as we seek conscience-based action to shape a new future for nursing and for health care.

"We call forth the passion of practicing nursing from this state of sovereignty and rightfully claim governance of our discipline. We call forth a repudiation of patterns that we create, or that are imposed upon us, that inhibit the full expression of our beings as nurses and persons. We call forth the opening of our hearts to reveal the prospects for action that carry us beyond the negative forces of passivity, contempt, frustration, cynicism, and despair; forces that keep us from living our wholeness and creating a world of peace and healing." (Cowling, Chinn, & Hagedorn, 2000, "Introduction")

The Connection Between Self-Care, Professional Self-Identity, and Self-Efficacy

Many of the factors discussed previously are interconnected. As Manojlovich (2007) writes, "Nurses' power may arise from three components: a workplace that has the requisite structures that promote empowerment; a psychological belief in one's ability to be empowered; and acknowledgement that there is power in the relationships and caring that nurses provide" ("Conclusion"). This last element of self-acknowledgement is directly related to a critical matter: *professional self-identity*.

Nurses need to know who they are so they can fully implement the BASE of Nursing (Potter, 2013) described in Chapter 1. Self-care (valuing) promotes self-identity (knowing), and a strong professional self-identity promotes self-efficacy (action).

According to Eisler (2002), a key aspect of self-care involves familiarizing oneself with components of domination/control and partnership/respect models. Once nurses can recognize domination patterns, they can consciously foster relationships based on partnership. This will not only make a huge difference for nurses—the ultimate benefit is that partnership-based relationships support co-creation of sustainable, environmentally friendly health care systems that work for everyone.

Partnership Exemplar: Nursing Salons

This chapter closes with a look at the importance of nurses coming together and supporting one another. Nurses practice professional self-care, increase professional identity, and promote issues that empower professional self-efficacy every time they participate in nursing professional organizations such as the American Nurses Association or the American Holistic Nurses Association. Another way to promote professional self-care is through nursing communities or movements that organize at the grassroots or local level. By nature, these communities often embody a partnership model with their flatter, less hierarchical organizational structure, facilitators rather than administrators, increased diversity, support for creativity, and empowerment of one another (Eisler & Montuori, 2001).

Nursing salons are a noteworthy example of a grassroots movement based on the partnership paradigm, and they are an innovative model of professional self-care. In 2001, nursing visionary Marie Manthey gathered a small group of nursing students and faculty to informally discuss their experiences in nursing. Manthey started with only six people, but the salon movement has grown to three or four monthly salons meeting in the Minneapolis/St. Paul area of Minnesota, as well as others that meet in California, Washington, Oregon, and England (Manthey, 2010). Each salon is a gathering of from 5–20 people. The event is very inclusive, with invitations spread by word of mouth or online. Dress is casual and dinner is provided. Guests only need to show up with a desire to talk about nursing. Manthey (2010) writes, "There is no formal agenda, and there are no minutes and no action steps—just a shared experience of touching the reality of nursing at a depth of meaning that enriches the practice and the experience of the participants" (p. 18).

Focused conversation begins during the meal when a facilitator asks, "What is on your mind about nursing tonight?" (Manthey, 2010). Each participant checks in and shares thoughts or issues related to nursing. Themes emerge during the check-in, and these become the topic of the evening. The evening closes with a checkout question that asks participants to respond to, "What is on your mind about nursing now?"

The nursing salons offer nurses an opportunity to do professional self-care. Through meeting and hearing the stories of other nurses, each nurse expands her/his understanding of professional self-identity. Manthey (2010) writes:

> *Novice nurses feel hope when they realize that seasoned staff nurses are still as passionate about nursing practice as they are. Veteran nurses feel the same hope as they see new nurses' depth of caring and passion about nursing. It becomes so clear to everyone that nursing is a culture, not just a job. (p. 19)*

Petty (2010), who regularly hosts nursing salons, reflects on the outcome of the salon experience:

> *Mostly, we have exposed our human sides and the intersection of ourselves with our practice; we have offered challenges and solutions and always more questions. Last and most important, we have reflected with the goal of making our practice and our profession better. (p. 189)*

Clearly, these salons, based on principles of partnership, empower self-efficacy and offer hope for the future of nursing.

AUTHOR'S EXPERIENCE OF A NURSING SALON

Before the door even opened, I could hear laughter and energetic conversation. I was greeted warmly by Marie Manthey and ushered in to meet a room full of nurses I did not previously know. We began with a meal prepared just for us— we did not need to cook. This genuine hospitality set the stage for a safe and meaningful conversation.

There are no hidden agendas in a salon, and everyone gets to speak. The conversation cannot be hijacked or monopolized because the structure of the dialog does not permit it. As we went around the room and listened intently to each person answer the question, "What is on your mind about nursing tonight?," several themes began to emerge. These themes guided the remaining dialogue. Like a well-orchestrated symphony, the evening concluded at an appointed time with one more summary go-around. The concluding comments reflected each of us had been moved by the experience of nurses sharing what is on our minds and hearts. – Teddie Potter

Conclusion

A partnership-based work environment fosters hierarchies of actualization where each employee is empowered to reach his or her full potential. In nursing, hierarchies of actualization are created when nurses are guaranteed professional sovereignty—including self-determined professional identity and self-governance or self-regulation of the profession. Furthermore, it is imperative that nurses be allowed to practice to the full extent of their education without domination and limitations imposed by other professions.

References

Americans for Nursing Shortage Relief Alliance (ANSR). (2012, March 29). Testimony of Americans for Nursing Shortage Relief (ANSR) Alliance regarding fiscal year 2013 appropriations for nursing workforce development programs and nurse managed health clinics. Retrieved from http://www.ansralliance.org/ANSR_FY2013_House_Testimony.pdf

Attridge, C. B. (1996). Analysis of powerlessness in nursing work. *Canadian Journal of Nursing Administration, 9*(2), 36-59.

Brehio, R. (2004). Survey shows workplace intimidation adversely affects patient safety. Retrieved from http://www.ismp.org/pressroom/pr20040331.pdf

Brown, T. (2011, May 7). Physician, heel thyself. *New York Times.* Retrieved from http://www.nytimes.com/2011/05/08/opinion/08Brown.html

Buerhaus, P. I., Auerbach, D. I., & Staiger, D. O. (2009). The recent surge in nurse employment: Causes and implications. *Health Affairs, 28*(4), w657w658.

Buresh, B., & Gordon, S. (2000). *From silence to voice: What nurses know and must communicate to the public.* Ithaca, NY: Cornell University Press.

Center for Partnership Studies. (n.d.). Organizational benefits of partnership systems. Retrieved from http://www.partnershipway.org/core-pathways/abcs-of-dominator-and-partnership-relations/two-social-possibilities-the-domination-system-and-the-partnership-system

Centers for Medicare and Medicaid Services. (2012). HCAHPS fact sheet. Retrieved from http://www.hcahpsonline.org/files/HCAHPS%20Fact%20Sheet%20May%202012.pdf

Coeling, H., & Cukr, P. (2000). Communication styles that promote perceptions of collaboration, quality, and nurse satisfaction. *Journal of Nursing Care Quality, 14*(2), 63-74.

Corley, M. C. (2002). Nurse moral distress: A proposed theory and research agenda. *Nursing Ethics, 9*(6), 636–650.

Cowling, R., Chinn, P.L., & Hagedorn, S. (2000). The nurse manifesto. Retrieved from http://www.nursemanifest.com

Droppleman, P. G., & Thomas, S. P. (1996). Anger in nurses: Don't lose it. Use it. *American Journal of Nursing, 96*(4), 26-32.

Edward, K. L., & Hercelinskyj, G. (2007). Burnout in the caring nurse: Learning resilient behaviors. *British Journal of Nursing, 16*(4), 240-242.

Eisler, R. (2002). *The power of partnership: Seven relationships that will change your life.* Novato, CA: New World Library.

Eisler, R., & Montuori, A. (2001). The partnership organization: A systems approach. *OD Practitioner, 33*(2), 11-17.

Epstein, E. G., & Delgado, S. (2010). Understanding and addressing moral distress. *OJIN: The Online Journal of Issues in Nursing, 15*(3). doi: 10.3912/OJIN. Vol15No03Man01

Furst, C. M., Finto, D., Malouf-Todaro, N., Moore, C., Orr, D., Santos, J.,…Tipton, P. H. (2013). Changing times: Enhancing clinical practice through evolving technology. *MEDSURG Nursing, 22*(2), 131-134.

Garets, D., & Davis, M. (2005). Electronic patient records: EMRs and EHRs. *Healthcare Informatics Online.* Retrieved from http://www.providersedge.com/ehdocs/ehr_articles/Electronic_Patient_Records-EMRs_and_EHRs.pdf

Institute of Medicine (IOM). (2003). *Key capabilities of an electronic health record system: Letter report.* Washington, DC: National Academies Press.

Institute of Medicine (IOM). (2010). *The future of nursing: Leading change, advancing health.* Washington, DC: National Academies Press.

Jaret, P. (2013, January 14). Mining electronic health records for revealing health data. *New York Times.* Retrieved from http://www.nytimes.com/2013/01/15/health/mining-electronic-records-for-revealing-health-data.html?_r=0

Jennings, B. M. (2008). Work stress and burnout among nurses: Role of the work environment and working conditions. In R. G. Hughes (Ed.), *Patient Safety and Quality: An Evidence-Based Handbook for Nurses* (pp. 137-158). Rockville, MD: Agency for Healthcare Research and Quality.

Laschinger, H., Finegan, J., & Shamian, J. (2001). Promoting nurses' health: Effect of empowerment on job strain and work satisfaction. *Nursing Economic$, 19*(2), 42-52.

Leape, L., Berwick, D., Clancy, C., Conway, J., Gluck, P., Guest, J.,...Isaac, T. (2009). Transforming healthcare: A safety imperative. *Quality Safety Health Care, 18*(6), 424-428. doi: 10.1136/qshc.2009.036954

Manderino, M. A., & Berkey, N. (1997). Verbal abuse of staff nurses by physicians. *Journal of Professional Nursing, 13*(1), 48-55.

Manojlovich, M. (2005a). Linking the practice environment to nurses' job satisfaction through nurse-physician communication. *Journal of Nursing Scholarship, 37*(4), 367-373.

Manojlovich, M. (2005b). Promoting nurses' self-efficacy: A leadership strategy to improve practice. *JONA, 35*(5), 271-278.

Manojlovich, M. (2007). Power and empowerment in nursing: Looking backward to inform the future. *OJIN: The Online Journal of Issues in Nursing, 12*(1). doi: 10.3912/OJIN.Vol12No01Man01

Manthey, M. (2010). A new model of healing for the profession of nursing. *Creative Nursing, 16*(1), 18-20.

Menachemi, N., & Collum, T. H. (2011). Benefits and drawbacks of electronic health record systems. *Risk Management and Healthcare Policy, 4*, 47-55.

Page, A. (Ed.). (2004). *Keeping patients safe: Transforming the work environment of nurses*. Washington, DC: National Academies Press.

Pendry, P. S. (2007). Moral distress: Recognizing it to retain nurses. *Nursing Economic$, 25*(4), 217-221.

Petty, M. (2010). Nursing salons: An opportunity to reflect on our practice. *Creative Nursing, 16*(4), 188-189.

Potter, T. M. (2013). *The BASE of nursing*. Unpublished manuscript, School of Nursing, University of Minnesota, United States of America.

Rosenstein, A. H. (2002). Nurse-physician relationships: Impact on nurse satisfaction and retention. *AJN, 102*(6), 26-34.

Spreitzer, G. M. (1995). Psychological empowerment in the workplace: Dimensions, measurement, and validation. *Academy of Management Journal, 38*(5), 1442-1465.

Wang, G., & Lee, P. D. (2009). Psychological empowerment and job satisfaction. *Group and Organization Management, 34*(3), 271-296.

Zuzelo, P. R. (2007). Exploring the moral distress of registered nurses. *Nursing Ethics, 14*(3), 344-359.

Chapter 8

Patient Care from a Domination and Partnership Perspective

"Care is the essence and the central unifying domain to characterize nursing."

–Leininger, 1988, p. 3

While most nurses acknowledge that care is the essence of nursing, the delivery of care can differ depending on whether it comes from a domination or partnership paradigm. This chapter provides concrete examples of these two different ways of relating to help nurses recognize domination when they see or hear it—in themselves, others, or institutional policies. Only in recognizing domination can you avoid it. If you do not see it, you can unintentionally promote systems that keep domination alive.

In the prologue to her book *Tomorrow's Children,* Eisler (2000) writes:

The partnership and dominator models not only describe individual relationships ... they describe systems of belief and social structures

*that either nurture and support—or inhibit and undermine—
equitable, democratic, nonviolent, and caring relations. Without an
understanding of these configurations—and the kind of education
that creates and replicates each—we unwittingly reinforce
structures and beliefs that maintain the inequitable, undemocratic,
violent, and uncaring relations which breed pathologies that afflict
and distort the human spirit and are today decimating our natural
habitat. (Prologue)*

In other words, from a very early age, the domination perspective becomes
part of our assumptions, our language, and our behaviors. Therefore, it is very
difficult for us to see, much less enact, an alternative model of behavior.

The Domination Perspective

Many nurses may think, "I know that I have experienced domination, but I am
not a dominator. I care about people, so I am a partner." But as you look at the
following scenarios, we invite you to ask yourself: Have I heard my colleagues
communicate this way? Have I spoken this way to patients or families?

Communication With a Patient: A Domination Approach

NURSE: "Hello, Mrs. Patterson, I am Sarah. I will be your nurse
today. I know that your son is visiting, but I need to take your
vitals and do your treatments. Then he can come back in, and you
can continue your conversation."

PATIENT: "I just don't feel like getting out of bed today."

NURSE: "We all have days like that; as a matter of fact I didn't
want to get out of bed today, either! But you need to follow the
orders from physical therapy, or you will not get stronger."

PATIENT: "I just can't seem to get better no matter what I do."

NURSE: (Placing her hands on her hips and shaking her head) "Well, one of the reasons you keep being readmitted to the hospital is because you do not follow the diabetic diet your doctor has ordered for you. I remember when you were in before. We did very thorough diabetic teaching, and here you are, back again!"

PATIENT: "Sometimes it is just so difficult to make changes when no one else in the family has to eat a special diet."

NURSE: "That 'special diet' that has been ordered for you can save your life. Don't you know we are trying to help?" (The nurse looks at her patient even more severely.) "I noticed candy bars in your bedside drawer. Why are you eating candy when your blood sugars keep getting out of control?"

PATIENT: (Defensively) "I just keep the candy there for my grandkids when they come to visit."

NURSE: "Well, I think I should lock the candy up at the nursing station, and you can ask us for it when your grandkids come. We don't want to see any more blood sugar spikes, do we?"

Of course, this kind of blaming, shaming, and talking down to someone who is being cared for is not confined to relationships between nurses and patients. As Eisler (2002) notes, it is often found between parents and children, teachers and students, and others.

But can you see these patterns of domination?

- The assumption that it is normal and right for one person to control another

- The assumption that authority should not be challenged

- The linking of care with control, even coercion

- The blaming and threatening of those with less power

- The norm of the physician giving *orders*, the nurse implementing the *orders*, and the patient expected to obey the *orders* without question

In short, though the nurse may have the best intentions, she exhibits a patronizing, condescending attitude, viewing her role as that of a superior ensuring compliance from an inferior.

Communication With a Nursing Assistant: A Domination Approach

Can nursing assistants (CNAs), housekeepers, dietary assistants, or health unit coordinators (HUCs) on your unit or in your institution give examples of times they have felt dominated and diminished by nursing colleagues? Listen for patterns of domination in the following conversation between Sam, the CNA, and Mary, the nurse:

> CNA: "Mary?"
>
> NURSE: "What is it? Can't you see I am busy? All these disruptions keep me from getting out on time."
>
> CNA: "I think you should come see Mrs. Jones. She's acting different from yesterday."
>
> NURSE: "Don't worry; she's just having a tough day."
>
> CNA: "It's just that when I gave her a shower her skin looked different."
>
> NURSE: "I know that you don't know much about cancer, but it's common for people to have a different look to them when they are getting treatments."
>
> CNA: (Sighs heavily.)
>
> NURSE: "Let me know if you see any *important* changes."

Did you hear the patterns of domination? They include:

- Authoritarian and inequitable social structure
- Rigid hierarchies
- Those in power suppress disagreements and conflicts

- Condescending pattern of communication

- Minimizing another person's concerns or dismissing his or her observations

- Blaming others—especially those with less power

- Assuming those with less power are also less intelligent

Many negative ramifications occur when health care relationships are based on the domination paradigm. When unlicensed assistive personnel (for example, nursing assistants) experience condescending communication and dominating behaviors from nurses, they are less likely to share timely, essential observations of early status changes. That delay can have very negative effects on patient health outcomes, as well as directly impact patient satisfaction. Similarly, patients may feel that their words and actions do not matter when the things they say are dismissed or disregarded. This again has negative impact, not only on patient satisfaction, but on obtaining vital information from patients. Indeed, if we do not pay attention to what patients tell us, why should they get involved in their own health care?

That is not all. When care providers dominate patients, patients may experience feelings of shame and humiliation, and these feelings may later prevent them from seeking care before they are in a critical state. This pattern, too, has negative implications for health outcomes and health care costs. In the same way, when families feel excluded or disregarded, nurses lose potential allies who can provide important health information and support to help improve the client's health behaviors.

COMMUNICATION WITH FAMILIES: A DOMINATION APPROACH

"Trust us. We'll let you know when there is something you need to know."

"Your husband has a health care directive. We will follow all his wishes and only ask for your involvement if we have a question."

"Your son's cares must be handled on a very strict schedule that you will need to follow. If you don't follow our orders, he'll end up right back in here, and then he'll have to be transferred to a nursing home where they can care for him appropriately."

Patient Care Given From the Partnership Perspective

Contrasting the partnership and domination perspectives, Eisler (n.d.) writes:

> *The* partnership system *supports mutually respectful and caring relations. Because there is no need to maintain rigid rankings of control, there is also no built-in need for abuse and violence. Partnership relations free our innate capacity to feel joy, to play. They enable us to grow mentally, emotionally, and spiritually. This is true for individuals, families, and whole societies. Conflict is an opportunity to learn and to be creative, and power is exercised in ways that empower rather than disempower others. (para. 3)*

Now see what the scenarios described previously in this chapter would look like when care is delivered from a partnership perspective.

Communication With a Patient: A Partnership Approach

NURSE: "Hello, Mrs. Patterson, I am Sarah. I will be your nurse today. I noticed that your son is visiting. Is this a good time to take your vital signs and do your treatments? Your son can watch and learn more about your treatments. He may be helping you when you go home, and that way he can ask questions. Would that be okay with you?"

PATIENT: "Yes, but I just don't feel like getting out of bed today."

NURSE: "I am sorry to hear that. Can you tell me how you are feeling? I know you have physical therapy scheduled. Can we work together on a plan so you feel like walking?"

PATIENT: "I just can't seem to get better no matter what I do."

NURSE: (Squeezing her patient's hand.) "I am sorry things are so difficult for you. You have tried things and it must be frustrating to have to come back into the hospital so often. We are here to work with you and support you as you learn how to manage your diabetes."

PATIENT: "Sometimes it is just so difficult to make changes when no one else in the family has to eat a special diet."

NURSE: "Eating is very personal, and it is difficult to have to change when we have patterns that are meaningful. Eating is also tied to social time and time as a family, so having to make changes feels like we are also making changes to family time. That is one reason I think it will be really helpful for you, your son, and me to talk about eating and how to stabilize your blood sugars ... By the way, I am wondering about something: I noticed candy bars in your bedside drawer."

PATIENT: "I keep the candy there for my grandkids when they come to visit."

NURSE: "I wonder, just so you're not tempted, would you like me to keep them in the nurse's station for when they come? That might also help your family understand how important your diet is for your health."

PATIENT: "No, I will explain it to them myself."

NURSE: "Great idea. Sometimes it is easier for patients to make changes in their diet when the whole family understands and supports your new diet. Do you think it would be helpful to have a family care conference where we talk about diabetes and how all of us can work together to keep you safe and healthy?"

PATIENT: "That would be nice. I won't feel so alone."

Did you hear the patterns of partnership? They include:

- Democratic and equitable social structure

- *Hierarchies of actualization*, where power is used to lift up and empower

- Mutual respect and trust without threats or blame

- High value placed on empathy and caring

- Conflict is used to creatively arrive at solutions

Communication With a Nursing Assistant: A Partnership Approach

CNA: "Mary?"

NURSE: "Yes?"

CNA: "I think you should come see Mrs. Jones. She's acting different from yesterday."

NURSE: "Can you describe what you are seeing?"

CNA: "It's just that when I gave her a shower, her skin looked different."

NURSE: "It could be related to the treatments she just started. Sometime the skin appears more pale or dusky. I really appreciate you letting me know, because something else might be going on. I'll come and take a look."

CNA: "Can I come with you?"

NURSE: "Sure! We are a team!"

CNA: "Thanks! I'd like to know what I should be looking for. I'm thinking of becoming a nurse one day."

Did you hear the patterns of partnership? They include:

- Democratic and equitable social structure

- Hierarchies of actualization

- Supportive and respectful patterns of communication

- Trusting that others are doing their best

- Assuming those with less power may have very important observations and insights

Partnership relations and structures have many benefits. Patient outcomes improve when health care relationships are based on the partnership paradigm. Patients feel encouraged to share their feelings, fears, and hopes for health. They are treated like partners, so they respond as partners, sharing important data and taking responsibility for their part in healing. When patients feel part of a team effort, they are more likely to seek care from a primary care provider than an emergency department staff they do not know. Again, early and consistent care offers the best chance for positive health outcomes and cost-effective treatments.

When families are treated like partners, they know how to be supportive of patients or clients as they recover from an acute condition or try to live with a chronic illness. Families who are partners are not afraid to call with status changes or to report treatment plans that do not appear effective.

COMMUNICATION WITH FAMILIES: A PARTNERSHIP APPROACH

"It is very important that you have all the information we have so we will update you regularly."

"We have your husband's health care directives. Let's go over them so we can be sure your family understands his decisions. You can ask us all the questions you need to."

"When your son returns home, you will be the primary caregivers. We will discuss the typical schedule we have had in the hospital and see how it can be modified to align with your patterns at home."

Similarly, when unlicensed assistive personnel (for example, nursing assistants) are treated as a valuable member of the health care team, they can feel more engaged and positive about their work. Another benefit from this partnership approach is less personnel turnover (Cready, Yeatts, Gosdin, & Potts, 2008). In addition, Hospital Consumer Assessment of Healthcare Providers and Systems (HCAHPS) scores may improve when hospital staff show increased responsiveness to patients' needs (Agency for Healthcare Research and Quality, 2012).

In short, partnership relations are foundational to better health care.

The Partnership Paradigm

Some readers might be wondering why Eisler's theories are necessary when health care is already beginning to recognize some of the benefits of partnership relationships. Actually, Eisler's domination/partnership framework (1987, 2002, 2007) is essential if we are to make lasting progress.

For example, Kou et al. (2012) note that:

- Families desire partnership and joint decision-making, but do not necessarily want the increased responsibility and autonomy that come with them.

- Reimbursement structures do not build in time for partnerships.

- People do not know how to be partners.

In *Partnering with Patients and Families to Design a Patient- and Family-Centered Health Care System: A Roadmap for the Future,* Conway et al. (2006) identified significant attitudinal, educational, and organizational barriers to better health care. Some of the barriers mentioned include:

- Providers "fear that patients' and families' suggestions will be unreasonable."

- Providers believe "that patient- and family-centered care is not necessary ('We are knowledgeable, caring professionals; we know what's best for our patients.')."

- Providers assume that "their patients are too poor, too violent, too un-educated, or too humble to be engaged or to engage."

- Overall there is a "[l]ack of understanding and skills for collaboration on the part of health care professionals and administrators as well as of patients and families."

- There is a "[t]endency to implement a top-down approach to initiating partnerships with insufficient effort put in to building staff commitment...."

- Alternately, there is a "tendency to implement a grassroots effort that lacks leadership commitment and support" (p. 30).

All these challenges can be directly traced to beliefs and assumptions associated with systems of domination. If we fail to identify domination, by default, it is allowed to persist. It is not enough, therefore, to invite patients and families to be full partners with health care providers. Patients, families, and providers must also be taught how to recognize, and then undo or dismantle, the domination thinking they have been socialized to accept as normal.

Health systems also need to aggressively challenge domination patterns found in health policies and systems of reimbursement. Indeed, as detailed in Chapter 13, health care does not exist in isolation from larger economic systems—which are, in turn, deeply embedded in social systems. And social systems are very different depending on the degree they orient to either end of the partnership/domination continuum.

Building a system based on the partnership model requires that we pay attention to the culture of our institutions and the values they support. Moreover, we have to pay attention to the organizational structure within which we operate, including the behaviors they encourage (or, alternately, discourage). This is why understanding the contrasting configurations of the domination model and the partnership model described in Chapter 3 is so important.

Eisler (as cited in Mercanti, 2012) talks about the importance of starting to build partnership systems from the foundation. She states:

> *You would not try to build a house without a plan or blueprint of the whole house—including its foundations. In the same way, we need the social blueprint of the partnership configuration to build a more equitable, caring, and sustainable future. And here too we have to pay particular attention to building its foundation in the formative relations that are the models (of either partnership or domination) that children first learn. (p. 145)*

Eisler recommends starting to build partnership systems at the most basic social unit. In health care that means beginning with the patient. In other words, to build a more effective health care system, we need to use partnership principles at the foundation: the point of delivery of patient care.

Seeds of domination are planted early and deep—so deep, in fact, that they are often difficult to detect and even more difficult to acknowledge. Therefore, all the employees of an organization need to work as partners, committed to the same goal of shifting assumptions, words, and actions. But "calling out" threads of domination cannot be done with shame or fear; it must be done with a deep commitment to continuous quality improvement and building a better system that works for everyone.

This is a very important point: Eisler (2002) emphasizes that blaming and shaming people, including ourselves, for old dysfunctional behaviors is yet another form of domination. Certainly we want to help others, as well as ourselves, identify and try to unlearn patterns of domination. But at the same time, do not hold yourself or others to impossible standards of perfection. Rather, treat others and yourself with the care and respect you would like to receive. That reinforces partnership behaviors and changes the organizational culture and structure in a partnership direction.

RESPECTFUL, NONDOMINATING BEHAVIORS IN THE WORKPLACE

Greet and acknowledge everyone you encounter no matter what position they hold.

Communicate gratitude and give credit to workers who submit ideas suggesting an improvement for quality or safety.

When an important guest arrives, introduce everyone he or she encounters, not just those with higher positions.

Each year, encourage employees to complete an anonymous online survey that evaluates those in leadership.

If you are the leader, be alert for opportunities that will challenge and expand your employees to help them reach their highest potential.

Create a culture where there is zero tolerance for bullying and incivility.

In sum, greater awareness of how people relate to one another is the first, basic, step. As you become more aware of patterns of domination that you have learned to accept, you can shift your behaviors, and with this, the cultural climate in our institutions.

By offering a powerful new systemic analysis, Eisler provides the framework and resources to understand and overcome the entrenched patterns of domination that stand in the way of a health care system that works for everyone. Building this system will not be easy or quick. But as more of us— providers, patients, families, payers, and politicians—work together, we *can* co-create it.

Partnership Exemplar: Patient- and Family-Centered Care

It is encouraging that a number of important initiatives have emerged in the previous decades to support health care systems' movement toward the partnership model. One of these initiatives, patient-centered care (PCC), is an approach to health care decision-making that provides an excellent example of the themes discussed in this chapter.

As you saw in the story of nursing (Chapters 4 and 5), PCC is not a new philosophy. However, the widespread *adoption* of this paradigm across health care *is* new. Also new—the fact that many experts now recognize that the involvement of patients in their own health care holds tremendous potential:

> As a philosophy of care, [family-centered care] (FCC), and the related term patient-centered care (PCC), have been recognized by multiple medical societies, health care systems, state and federal legislative bodies, the Institute of Medicine, and Healthy People 2020 as integral to patient health, satisfaction, and health care quality. (Kuo et al., 2012, p. 297)

Along with this recognition of the value of patient-centered care, health care providers and policymakers are beginning to shift from a domination model of patient care to a partnership model. For example, prior to the 1980s and 1990s, hospitalized children were often isolated from their families by hierarchies of domination that maintained strict visiting hours and rigid rules around family and sibling visits. Likewise, it was not uncommon for children with intellectual limitations or chronic health conditions to be institutionalized. Eventually, however, research demonstrated the traumatic implications for pediatric patients when isolated from their families.

Care delivery models began changing in a partnership direction (Jolley & Shields, 2009). For example, a policy statement issued by the American Academy of Pediatrics (2012) summarizes findings on the benefits of patient- and family-centered care (PFCC):

- Improved patient and family outcomes;

- Improved patient and family experience of care;

- Increased patient and family satisfaction;

- Increased professional satisfaction; and

- Decreased health care costs, leading to more effective use of health care resources. (p. 397)

Family-centered care principles can now also be measured within organizations. These agreed-upon principles include information sharing, respect, honoring differences, partnership and collaboration, negotiation, and care in the context of family and community (Kuo et al., 2012). All this signals movement toward partnership-based, family-centered health care becoming a benchmark for excellence for highly effective health care organizations (Institute of Medicine [IOM], 2001; Kuo et al., 2012; Leape et al., 2009). Equally significant is that a growing number of organizations are championing this approach, as illustrated by the example described next.

The Institute for Patient- and Family-Centered Care

In 1992, the nonprofit organization Institute for Patient- and Family-Centered Care (IPFCC) was initiated. Through research, education, consultation, strategic partnership development, and information dissemination, the organization seeks to fulfill the following vision:

> *We at the Institute envision a profound change in the way health care is provided to individuals and their families. In every encounter, health and human service professionals will seek to build on the strengths of patients and families, enhancing their confidence and competence. The health care delivery system will recognize and encourage patient and family strengths, choice, and independence. (IPFCC, 2011, "About Us" section)*

The IPFCC is a champion for patient- and family centered care for all health care consumers, of all ages, in all settings. It also advocates for patient- and family-centered policies at state and federal levels (Johnson et al., 2008).

The IPFCC took the core concepts of FCC and expanded them:

- **Respect and dignity.** Health care practitioners listen to and honor patient and family perspectives and choices. Patient and family knowledge, values, beliefs, and cultural backgrounds are incorporated into the planning and delivery of care.

- **Information Sharing.** Health care practitioners communicate and share complete and unbiased information with patients and families in ways that are affirming and useful. Patients and families receive timely, complete, and accurate information in order to effectively participate in care and decision-making.

- **Participation.** Patients and families are encouraged and supported in participating in care and decision-making at the level they choose.

- **Collaboration.** Patients and families are also included on an institution-wide basis. Health care leaders collaborate with patients and families in policy and program development, implementation, and evaluation; in health care facility design; and in professional education, as well as in the delivery of care. (IPFCC, 2010a, "FAQ" section)

Most providers today are willing to collaborate on treatment plans with patients, but the IPFCC invites providers and health systems to integrate partnership with patients through every level of the health care system. By inviting patients and families to participate in areas that were previously the domain of those with the most power (for example, policy decisions and professional education), the IPFCC promotes true partnership-based systems of health.

In order to implement a system-wide PFCC approach, the IPFCC recommends providers, unit managers, and health system executives start by assessing an organization's culture. The IPFCC (2010b) publishes an excellent self-reflection tool called "A Checklist for Attitudes about Patients and Families as Advisors"; it appears in Figure 8.1. This tool guides individuals to deeply reflect on assumptions and beliefs that can block PCC and FCC programs.

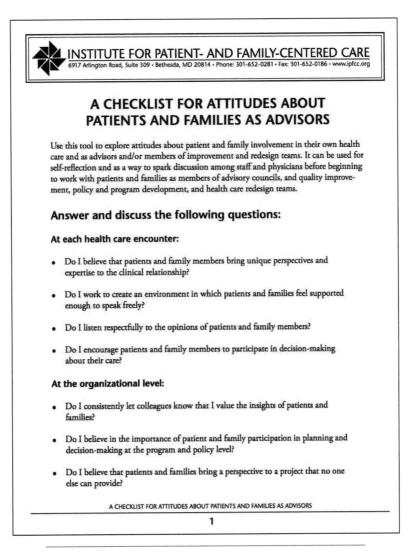

FIGURE 8.1: A CHECKLIST FOR ATTITUDES ABOUT
PATIENTS AND FAMILIES AS ADVISORS.

*Reprinted with permission from the Institute for Patient-
and Family-Centered Care: www.ipfcc.org*

Once individuals are aware of their own beliefs and attitudes, they can more effectively assess the culture of their work environment. The IPFCC (2010c) assessment tool entitled "Are Families Considered Visitors in Our Hospital or Unit?" Figure 8.2 shows this tool, which allows individual care providers, managers, and health care executives to explore the degree to which their organization is patient- and family-centered in its care.

INSTITUTE FOR PATIENT- AND FAMILY-CENTERED CARE
6917 Arlington Road, Suite 309 • Bethesda, MD 20814 • Phone: 301-652-0281 • Fax: 301-652-0186 • www.ipfcc.org

ARE FAMILIES CONSIDERED VISITORS IN OUR HOSPITAL OR UNIT?

In advancing the practice of family-centered care—changing the concept of families as visitors and recognizing families as partners in the care of patients—it is important to examine staff practices and the infrastructure of a hospital to determine how well family presence and participation is supported. This checklist may be useful in understanding current policies and practices and prioritizing action steps for a plan for change.

	Yes	No	Perceived Priority for Change

▼ Philosophy of Care

	Yes	No	Perceived Priority for Change
Does the philosophy of care statement for the hospital or unit acknowledge the importance of families to the care and comfort of patients?	☐	☐	1 2 3
Were patients and families involved in developing the philosophy of care statement?	☐	☐	1 2 3

▼ Policies

	Yes	No	Perceived Priority for Change
In written policies, is there acknowledgment of varied family structures and composition, and an acknowledgment of a patient's right to self-define family?	☐	☐	1 2 3
In written policies, is there a distinction made between *families* (however family is defined by the patient) and *visitors*, those friends, colleagues, or distant relatives who may wish to visit the patient or the patient's family?	☐	☐	1 2 3
Are policies regarding family presence and participation written as guidelines to foster flexibility and the individualization of staff practices to each patient's priorities and preferences?	☐	☐	1 2 3
Do hospital or unit guidelines (or policies) welcome families 24 hours a day, even during rounds, shift changes, a code, or emergency situations?	☐	☐	1 2 3

Source: Ahmann, E., Abraham, M.R. & Johnson, B.H. (2003). *Changing the Concept of Families as Visitors: Supporting Family Presence and Participation*. Bethesda, MD: Institute for Family-Centered Care.

This checklist has been adapted from other self-assessment inventories developed by the Institute for Family-Centered Care. Additional checklists are included in each of the Pinwheel Series publications produced by the Institute for Family-Centered Care.

ARE FAMILIES CONSIDERED VISITORS IN OUR HOSPITAL OR UNIT?

1

FIGURE 8.2: ARE FAMILIES CONSIDERED VISITORS IN OUR HOSPITAL OR UNIT?

Reprinted with permission from the Institute for Patient- and Family-Centered Care: www.ipfcc.org

The core values of partnership—power *with* rather than *over*, hierarchies of actualization, respectful communication, shared decision-making, and encouragement of creativity and innovation—are clearly embedded throughout the IPFCC's mission, vision, initiatives, and education materials.

Conclusion

It is politically correct for providers and institutions to claim they offer patient-centered care, but for most this simply means that the care is centered or focused on the patient. The patient is little more than a passive recipient of plans developed around them and without their input. The only way authentic patient- and family-centered care will become manifest is when health care professionals fully embrace a partnership paradigm. When that happens, we will see patients and families participating as full partners in care conferences, in the education of health professionals, and in the design of health care policy.

References

Agency for Healthcare Research and Quality. (2012). HCAHPS fact sheet. Retrieved from http://www.hcahpsonline.org/files/HCAHPS%20Fact%20Sheet%20May%20 2012.pdf

American Academy of Pediatrics. (2012). Patient- and family-centered care and the pediatrician's role. *Pediatrics, 129*(2), 394-404. doi: 10.1542/peds.2011-3084

Conway, J., Johnson, B., Edgman-Levitan, S., Schlucter, J., Ford, D., Sodomka, P., & Simmons, L. (2006). *Partnering with patients and families to design a patient- and family-centered health care system: A roadmap for the future.* Bethesda, MD: Institute for Family-Centered Care.

Cready, C. M., Yeatts, D. E., Gosdin, M. M., & Potts, H. F. (2008). CNA empowerment: Effect on job performance and work attitudes. *Journal of Gerontological Nursing, 34*(3), 26-35.

Eisler, R. (n.d.). Shifting our relationships from domination to partnership. Retrieved from http://www.partnershipway.org/core-pathways/abcs-of-dominator-and-partnership-relations/copy_of_partnership-relationships

Eisler, R. (1987). *The chalice and the blade: Our history, our future.* San Francisco, CA: HarperSanFrancisco.

Eisler, R. (2000). Excerpts from the prologue to *Tomorrow's Children.* Retrieved from http://www.partnershipway.org/learn-more/other-books-incorporating-partnership/ preview/excerpt-from-the-foreword-of-tomorrows-children

Eisler, R. (2002). *The power of partnership: Seven relationships that will change your life.* Novato, CA: New World Library.

Eisler, R. (2007). *The real wealth of nations: Creating a caring economics.* San Francisco, CA: Berett-Koehler.

Institute of Medicine (IOM). (2001). *Crossing the quality chasm: A new health system for the 21st century.* Washington, DC: National Academies Press.

Institute of Patient- and Family-Centered Care (IPFCC). (2010a). What are the core concepts of patient- and family centered care? Retrieved from http://www.ipfcc.org/ faq.html

Institute of Patient- and Family-Centered Care (IPFCC). (2010b). A checklist for attitudes about patients and families as advisors. Retrieved from http://www.ipfcc.org/tools/ downloads-tools.html

Institute of Patient- and Family-Centered Care (IPFCC). (2010c). Are families considered visitors in our hospital or unit? Retrieved from http://www.ipfcc.org/tools/ downloads-tools.html

Institute of Patient- and Family-Centered Care (IPFCC). (2011). About us. Retrieved from http://www.ipfcc.org/about/index.html

Johnson, B., Abraham, M., Conway, J., Simmons, L., Edgman-Levitan, S., Sodomka, P.,...Ford, D. (2008). *Partnering with patients and families to design a patient- and family-centered health care system: Recommendations and promising practices.* Bethesda, MD: Institute for Patient- and Family Centered Care.

Jolley, J., & Shields, L. (2009). The evolution of family centered care. *Journal of Pediatric Nursing, 24*(2), 164-170.

Kuo, D. Z., Houtrow, A. J., Arango, P., Kuhlthau, K. A., Simmons, J. M., & Neff, J. M. (2012). Family-centered care: Current applications and future directions in pediatric health care. *Maternal Child Health Journal, 16*(2), 297-305.

Leape, L., Berwick, D., Clancy, C., Conway, J., Gluck, P., Guest, J.,...Isaac, T. (2009). Transforming healthcare: A safety imperative. *Quality Safety Health Care, 18*(6), 424-428. doi: 10.1136/qshc.2009.036954

Leininger, M. M. (Ed.). (1988). *Care: The essence of nursing and health*. Detroit, MI: Wayne State University Press.

Mercanti, S. (2012). In conversation with Riane Eisler. *Le Simplegadi, 10,* 143-154. Retrieved from http://all.uniud.it/simplegadi

Chapter 9
Partnership-Based Intraprofessional Relationships

"Nurses eat their young."

–Author unknown

NURSES EAT THEIR YOUNG

A nursing student came to my office and broke into tears as she recounted her experience out at clinicals. All her life she had wanted to be a nurse in the military. She wanted to serve her country by serving people in some of the most challenging situations and most inhospitable settings. She was in her senior year and starting to look at various recruiting materials.

With pride she told her clinical preceptor that she felt her dream of becoming a military nurse was within reach.

The preceptor laughed and responded, "They won't take you. You're too fat."

With one deft blow, this nurse thoughtlessly erased the lifelong dream of a future nurse.

Why do abused people turn and abuse one another? From a purely basic level of survival, this does not seem to make sense. Or does it? The answer lies in whether you live according to partnership or domination values.

This chapter explores the rather common phenomenon of nurse bullying, or *lateral violence*, and identifies the domination forces that call it into play. Once you understand how the domination system promotes and fosters incivility, you can consciously choose a different path.

As discussed in previous chapters, nurses share similar responses to oppression in the workplace, including moral distress; disengagement from patient care; increased frequency of sick days, depression, substance abuse, and medication errors; decreased immunity; and early attrition from the field of nursing (Bartholomew, 2006). Nursing literature also acknowledges another adverse response to oppression: bullying or lateral violence (LV). "Lateral violence refers to acts that occur between colleagues, where bullying is described as acts perpetrated by one in a higher level of authority and occur over time" (American Nurses Association [ANA], 2011).

No one likes to admit bad behavior, but the nursing profession must understand and confront this harmful pattern. Lateral violence and bullying are symptoms related to domination systems. By recognizing the symptom, nurses can address the root cause and move to a healthier place in our relationships with one another.

Identifying Patterns of Domination

Rigid professional hierarchies, dysfunctional communication from providers, technology that decreases the amount of time nurses can spend with patients, and external pressures to increase services with fewer resources all contribute to the creation of an oppressive work environment.

Verbal abuse is probably the most common form of incivility in health care (ANA, 2011; Institute for Safe Medication Practices [ISMP], 2004). Rowe and Sherlock (2005) surveyed over 213 hospital nurses about their experiences with verbal abuse in the workplace. Their findings demonstrated that nurses themselves perpetuate systems of domination.

In considering the different sources of verbal abuse a nurse can experience, Rowe and Sherlock (2005) found:

The most frequent source of abuse was nurses (27%), followed by patients' families (25%), doctors (22%), patients (17%), residents (4%), other (3%) and interns (2%). Of those who selected a nurse as the most frequent source, staff nurses were reported to be the most frequent nursing source (80%) followed by nurse managers (20%). (p. 242)

This study shows that the greatest number of incidents come not from physicians, but from fellow nurses. Moreover, it indicates that nurses who have the least power are the most likely to experience verbal abuse. These findings have significant implications for the profession, especially given the connection between the oppression of care providers, their dysfunctional coping responses, and the impact this has on patient outcomes.

Lateral violence has emerged as a recognized phenomenon in nursing. Embree and White (2010) synthesized the literature on lateral violence and found that lateral violence is understood to mean nurse-to-nurse aggression that includes verbal, physical, or emotional abuse, and a consistent behavior pattern designed to control or devalue a peer (p. 168). They also found that causes of lateral violence include the following:

- Role issues

- Oppression

- Strict hierarchies

- Disenfranchising work practices

- Low self-esteem

- Perception of powerlessness (Embree & White, 2010, p. 166)

As previously noted, all of these behaviors are directly connected to systems of domination and oppression.

Renowned Brazilian education philosopher Paulo Freire (1993) focused his research on oppressed groups and found that oppressed groups themselves tend to exhibit certain oppressive behaviors. These *oppressed group behaviors* (OGBs) include identification with the oppressor, conformity, horizontal [lateral] violence, self-deprecation, and emotional dependence. Freire also found that these destructive behaviors are handed down from generation to generation, as people do not realize there is any other alternative. This phenomenon is exemplified by the tendency of many nurses to accept without questioning the phrase "Nurses eat their young."

Daiski (2004) interviewed 20 staff nurses to examine the nature of intra-nursing relationships. She found that rigid hierarchies and mutual lack of support were often the norm. Furthermore, "Both types of relationships were found to be inextricably linked, sustaining nurses' oppression through disempowering discourses" (p. 43).

This finding supports Freire's theory that oppressed groups participate in maintaining systems of oppression—including their own. The first theorist to apply Freire's theory to nursing was Roberts (1983; 2000), who proposed that nurses manifest behaviors common to oppressed groups. Roberts (2000) wrote:

> *Powerless groups have difficulty taking control of their own destiny because internalized beliefs about their own inferiority lead to a cycle of self-hatred and inability to unite to challenge the inequality of power. Empowerment of these groups involves the development of a more positive self-image through understanding of the cycle.* (p. 71)

As discussed in Chapter 7, self-care promotes positive professional self-identity, and positive self-identity plays a significant role in self-efficacy and the ability to be effective partners in systems change. These factors need to be in place before there can be a decrease in episodes of lateral violence.

Similarly, Daiski (2004) recommended that the profession of nursing needs to be an active advocate of creating systemic changes that promote healthier environments. She writes:

Change for the better needs to come from within the nursing profession. To develop effective strategies, bedside nurses have to be included in decision-making processes affecting them and their practice, about which they are the experts. Mutual respect, awareness-raising through education, development of caring nursing communities, mentorship and non-hierarchical leadership are key to stopping dis-empowering discourses and practices amongst nurses. (p. 43)

Using the BASE of Nursing to Address Lateral Violence

As noted throughout this book, it is difficult—if not impossible—to maintain partnership models when systems of domination go unchallenged. Therefore, in order for nurses to unify and become effective leaders of change, the profession must recognize and challenge patterns of domination wherever they are found.

The BASE of Nursing (Potter, 2013) offers the profession of nursing an effective way of challenging domination. Through empathic presence and deep listening to one another, frustrations related to working in a domination system are revealed through *narratives of oppression*. These stories contain the data that point to the root cause or source of the emotions that prompted the lateral violence. Once the root cause is understood, nurses can work together using best-practice methods and active caring to shift the system toward partnership.

- **Being Present:** Build a community in the workplace. Agree that behaviors of lateral violence are not acceptable. Support and nurture people when they experience domination.

- **Stories/Narrative-Based Evidence:** Encourage those who have been harmed by experiences of domination to tell their story. Sometimes simply telling the story allows people to discharge negative emotions that they may otherwise direct laterally at peers.

- **Evidence from Science:** Once an incident or ongoing process of oppression is "diagnosed," nurses have many best-practice resources that they can use to resolve specific issues. For example, both the ANA and Quality and Safety Education for Nurses (QSEN) describe the negative impact that oppression has on the profession and patient outcomes and offer excellent resources to help nurses address this issue. Similarly, the Center for Partnership Studies (n.d.) offers resources, interviews, videos, and education programs that nurses can use to address systems of domination (described in the websites www.partnershipway.org and www.caringeconomy.org).

- **Active Caring:** Several preventive measures and interventions can be applied to heal environments where lateral violence occurs. The following methods are suggested by the ANA (2011):

  - Not accepting violent or abusive behavior

  - Protecting victims from retribution after they report

  - Using assistance programs

  - Interrupting violent or abusive behavior

  - Assessing the unit and raising the awareness of colleagues

  - Considering solutions and encouraging dialogue

  - Creating unit-specific guidelines ("Solutions" section)

It may be helpful for nurses to know that they have many allies, from a wide variety of health care organizations, supporting efforts to transform their work environments. For example, Leape et al. (2009) representing the National Patient Safety Foundation, write:

Capturing the soul of an organization, where joy and meaning resides, requires a true partnership to align values among organization leaders, professionals and the workforce. Leaders must create the environment where it is possible for improvements to take place. However, the richest source of ideas for improvement is the frontline workers. It is they who live in the complexities of the current systems, have direct insights into failures and see daily opportunities for improvement. (p. 427)

Nurses do indeed live in the complexities of the current systems, and our presence, stories, and actions will help us create meaningful change.

Lateral Violence: A Partnership Solution

Eisler's work offers nurses an effective template for shifting systems from domination to partnership. She starts by revealing the realities of domination and the possibility of an alternative model based on partnership:

> *We are all familiar with these two models from our own lives. We know the pain, fear, and tension of relations based on domination and submission, on coercion and accommodation, of jockeying for control, of trying to manipulate and cajole when we are unable to express our real feelings and needs, of the miserable, awkward tug of war for that illusory moment of power rather than powerlessness, of our unfulfilled yearning for caring and mutuality, of all the misery, suffering, and lost lives and potentials that come from these kinds of relations. Most of us have also, at least intermittently, experienced another way of being, one where we feel safe and seen for who we truly are, where our essential humanity and that of others shines through, perhaps only for a little while, lifting our hearts and spirits, enfolding us in a sense that the world can after all be right, that we are valued and valuable. (Eisler, 2000, prologue to* Tomorrow's Children*)*

Eisler, writing for the Center for Partnership Studies, offers a road map for intentionally choosing partnership beliefs and behaviors rather than those that support domination. Eisler writes:

> *Before Newton identified gravity, apples fell off trees all the time but people had no name or explanation for what was happening. The partnership and domination systems not only give us names for different ways of relating but also an explanation for what lies behind these differences. (n.d.)*

Having an explanation for what is happening is critical for freeing nursing from the domination paradigm. However, once we are able to see domination, we need to have a proven process for challenging it. In *Tomorrow's Children: A Blueprint for Partnership Education in the 21ˢᵗ Century*, Eisler (2000) suggests four key actions:

1. "To build a partnership future, the people who populate that future—today's and tomorrow's children—must understand, experience, and value partnership" (p. 216).

    To accomplish this, the nursing profession can:

    -   Thread partnership theory and principles through nursing education curricula.

    -   Role-model partnership communication and behaviors for nursing students during their clinical rotations.

    -   Make a deep commitment to treat newly hired employees with respect and dignity.

2. "An equitable and peaceful future requires family, social, and political institutions based on partnership between the male and female halves of humanity" (p. 217).

    To accomplish this, the nursing profession can:

    -   Create safe places for unit nurses to discuss experiences of gender-based discrimination in their lives and/or work.

    -   Develop unit-specific ways to promote community and inclusivity.

    -   Recognize that within the nursing profession, traditional patterns of men over women may be reversed to women over men. Both of these patterns are dysfunctional.

3. "For a good quality of life, we need economic measures and systems of reward that encourage empathy, creativity, and give real value to caring for self, others, and nature" (p. 218).

To accomplish this, the nursing profession can:

- Participate in Eisler's Caring Economy Leadership Program (Caring Economy Campaign, 2011) and/or her Cultural Transformation Course. These programs are discussed further in Chapters 13 and 14.

- Make certain that all nurses are educated in principles of partnership and domination as well as caring economics so they can be articulate advocates and leaders in creating healthy systems of care.

- Reward innovation and creative solutions proposed by employees in all levels of the health care system.

4. "To build a partnership culture we need to reexamine beliefs, myths, and stories—strengthening those that promote partnership and discarding those that do not" (p. 219).

To accomplish this, the nursing profession can:

- Examine the language and assumptions embedded in nursing textbooks and other resources (Potter, 2010).

- Acknowledge and honor exemplars of partnership-based nursing at the unit level, the health organization level, and the national level. The American Academy of Nursing's (AAN) Raise the Voice Edge Runners provides role models for this action:

> *Nursing has the answer to the many problems that plague our health care system. Raise the Voice Edge Runners are practical innovators who have led the way in bringing new thinking and new methods to a wide range of health care challenges. Edge Runners have developed care models and interventions that demonstrate significant, sustained clinical and financial outcomes. Many of the stories underscore the courage and fighting spirit of nurse leaders who have persevered despite institutional inertia or resistance. (AAN, 2013)*

- Invite partnership-based nursing exemplars to be guest lecturers for nursing education courses, telling their personal stories of overcoming domination in favor of partnership.

The following interview is an example of this approach.

Partnership Exemplar: Marie Manthey and the History of Primary Nursing

Throughout the history of nursing, heroic nurses have risen up to meet powers of domination with powers of partnership. One recent exemplar is Marie Manthey, the cocreator of Primary Nursing.

Primary Nursing is a patient care delivery system that focuses on the therapeutic relationship between a patient and his or her identified primary nurse, who assumes responsibility for planning and coordinating the patient's care through the entire length of stay or health care event (Person, as cited in Koloroutis, 2004, p. 164). Primary Nursing started in 1969, on Station 32 at the University of Minnesota Hospital, and is now a model for nursing practice around the globe.

The following interview with Marie Manthey describes a stressful work environment similar to the one that many nurses experience today. Instead of turning to lateral violence and other *patterns of domination*, Manthey and others used partnership principles to create a new model of care that works for everyone (M. Manthey, personal communication, May 9, 2013).

> **Teddie Potter (TP):** Before we start your story, let's give our readers a little bit of context. How large was Station 32?
>
> **Marie Manthey (MM):** It was a 23-bed medical unit with tertiary care patients before medical ICUs.
>
> **TP:** And what was your staffing like?

MM: 6.0 registered nurses, 7.5 licensed practical nurses, 4.5 nursing assistants, and 1.5 ward clerks. Now that's 24-hours-a-day total staffing, which resulted in 2 RNs on days, 2 on evenings, and 1 on nights, when the component was full and didn't have a vacancy.

TP: Did your RNs have associate degrees or baccalaureate degrees?

MM: Diploma and baccalaureate.

TP: Prior to Primary Nursing, all of the nursing care was delivered using a team nursing model based on rigid hierarchies. Please share your story of the creation of Primary Nursing, a partnership-based model of care.

MM: We started on a unit where the staff was experiencing a great deal of frustration and anger because of changes that were being imposed upon them. Administration wanted us to be able to test things out on this unit, and then they would be implemented hospital-wide.

So we did a lot of things: change the way linen was distributed, change the distribution of medications, change the way pharmacy interacted, change the lab system, change the supply system. Before these changes, we did six studies in order to collect baseline data of what was actually happening in the operation of the unit.

We were not intending to change the delivery system. We didn't even think delivery systems at that time. I don't think anyone in the profession was thinking delivery systems.

We did want, however, to improve nursing practice. The thought was that by relieving nurses of non-nursing work, they would automatically spend more time at the bedside.

The evidence began to come in from other people who had been doing similar work. Using this approach did not increase the amount of time nurses were spending with patients. Then I reviewed a study that was done at the University of Iowa where they increased the professional staff by 60% and found no significant increase in the amount of time nurses were spending with patients.

They did a 3-week in-service to reacquaint the nurses with actual care, and there was even less time spent with patients after that. This finding forced us to look at the role of the RN.

We found the team leader role was so filled with mini-managerial functions that the nurses had very little time to actually interact with patients. In trying to reinforce the notion that care should be individualized to each patient, we created additional stress on an already change-weary staff. Eventually, the tension mounted, so that there was a threat of a mass resignation.

TP: How did you respond?

MM: We had a night meeting at my house. Absolutely radical, because I was an assistant director, and we had the aides and the orderlies and the LPNs and the RNs all at my house. And that never happened, across those kinds of ranks before. We served wine and drank beer and sat before the fireplace and just talked and talked and talked. And the nurses asked that night if they could stop being team leaders the next day, if they could just arrange assignments around where they felt their competence was and the way they wanted to utilize the support staff.

We said, "Okay." But we knew we didn't have the authority to do that. This was definitely a director of nursing authority thing because Team Nursing was required by the NLN for an accreditation of schools. So for us to be throwing away Team Nursing, even on one unit, was bringing high risk to the hospital and their relationship to the [University of Minnesota] School of Nursing.

Also, we didn't talk to the doctors; in fact, we didn't tell anyone what we were doing. Actually, we didn't yet have language to explain the changes.

I personally had a barrier to even communicating with the doctors, so I didn't. Once we had implemented this new model of nursing care delivery, we began to get comments back like, "I don't know what you're doing on [Station] 32, but it sure is nice." Comments like, "Did you get some more staff around here? Because it seems like you have more help."

And, of course, administration was just eating it up, but nursing supervisors were outraged.

TP: Why?

MM: They didn't know what was happening. Nobody had asked their permission, nobody had talked to them about it; they didn't know. And who were we anyway, to change things like that?

TP: [The director of nursing finally toured the unit to find out for herself what was happening on Station 32.] When she visited, what did she see?

MM: She saw people assuming responsibility, doing things without checking, checking, checking, checking, checking with somebody in charge, and doing total patient care. We had gone from the functional task of "The aides take the temperatures, the LPNs do the blood pressures, the RNs pass the meds," to the RN in the room doing the TPR, BP, medications, all in one fell swoop, with as much support from the LPNs as they needed for those tasks. So it was a very sensible arrangement.

TP: So, paint for us a picture of Team Nursing prior to Primary Nursing.

MM: There was always one RN in charge of each team. In the old days, she would get a report and then give a report, because the LPNs and the aides didn't listen to the same report as the RNs.

Team leaders actually had to learn to report at three different levels of language, which is so stupid, it's unbelievable.

And everything was transmitted again and again and again, which only raised all kinds of opportunities for errors. The nurse would give her report, and then she'd get her meds ready. And she was doing meds for the whole team, so the pouring and the passing of the meds would take a significant chunk of time, during which time she'd also be answering questions and dealing with any issues that were coming up. Her job was to make sure that people got to coffee on time and back on time, to lunch on time and back on time; that all the treatments were done; and she made rounds with the doctor. It was just run, run, run, run, run, run, run.

TP: So then what did you switch to? What was the new path?

MM: The new path was for the RN to have a caseload of three or four—maybe five—patients with an aide, perhaps, supporting her. The LPN would have the other three or four or five or six, with whatever kind of support was needed.

So they would just divide the patients among the staff, using the criteria that the best qualified person provided the clinical support needed for that particular patient.

And we would let LPNs do everything. We had them charting, we had them doing up to the extent of their license—which is today, even, a great rarity—to let people practice to the level of their license. The controls we think we have to put on people because we don't know how to manage them for success are just wasteful!

TP: I imagine under this new system, engagement, satisfaction with work, and a sense of meaning began to return to staff.

MM: There was also an increase in patient and doctor satisfaction.

TP: When nurses were able to practice in their full role, did you see things shift in their interprofessional relationships?

MM: Absolutely. A few weeks after [Primary Nursing] started, the admitting department called me and said, "What is going on in Station 32?" And I said, "Why? What's happening? Why are you asking?" (Because there were three medical units, all with the same medical staff and the same criteria for patients.)

[The admitting department replied that] "All of the doctors want their patients on Station 32 now. We keep getting these requests."

TP: Related to patient satisfaction?

MM: Because of increased patient satisfaction and good nursing care. It was such a total evolution of the nursing role. I was so aware of what was happening and how consistent it was with what we had read in school and what we all wanted to do. It was happening!

TP: Previously, nursing practice did not match nursing theory. This is often true today as well.

MM: Right.

TP: So really this is everything that partnership is about. Ideas come when you work together for a common good, when you support each other in hierarchies of actualization instead of hierarchies of domination. Partnership allows you to work with each other rather than against each other.

MM: [Yes, in domination] we live by the belief that people will screw up if given half a chance, and we need to set up mechanisms to control them.

I found it necessary to try to define the role of the primary nurse in the language of responsibility, authority, and accountability. That framework enabled me to explain to people how this role was different than the role of the team leader or any other role we had for nurses where the responsibility level was ambiguous or shared. So there was a lot of speaking in the early years about the difference between shared responsibility and clarification of total responsibility.

TP: People might not be familiar with Responsibility, Authority, Accountability (RAA)…

MM: Responsibility means being able to respond. There are two characteristics of it that are important. One is it needs to be clear. Lack of clarity is what leads to all kinds of dysfunction within a system.

TP: And we also know that lateral violence is correlated with lack of clarity.

MM: Right. So the second characteristic of responsibility is that it has to be accepted by the individual, and this is the key to self-management.

In my experience, I am thoroughly convinced that a failure to accept responsibility that has been legitimately allocated results in victim thinking and dependency.

I've seen nurses do all the tasks of primary care and going on interprofessional rounds with a primary physician, yet they're not functioning as primary nurses. Eventually, I came to realize the problem was nonacceptance of the responsibility. This was manifested by an unwillingness to establish the responsibility relationship with the patient or their family.

They don't have a sense of their own authority. So by establishing a relationship with their patients, nurses get in touch with the legitimate authority that they already have but they're not aware of.

TP: And this is a key ability or knowledge, as we move into interprofessional practice. If nurses don't know who they are, and they have not taken responsibility for what nurses bring to the table, they cannot practice as full partners. So that's responsibility. What comes next?

MM: Then authority comes. This is a word we don't use in nursing. Authority is power. Authority is the right to act in the areas which you have been allocated and have accepted responsibility.

Whatever you and the patient-partner agree on is the way things are going to be done. And, how are you going to carry out those agreed-upon actions? That is where the power comes from. We are woefully ignorant about the use of power.

TP: Well, we frequently don't teach about it in nursing school, and because power is often used against us, we shy away from it.

MM: That's right. I think authority is something we are neglecting within our profession. We don't use the right words; I think we should be using the word *authority*.

TP: That leads us back to the beginning of this book where we describe the unique medicine of nursing. When I realize I have a unique medicine, I have authority over that medicine. It's not something that somebody else can take away.

MM: That's right. We own it.

TP: And then accountability....

MM: The way I define it, it's the retrospective review of the work that was done to determine whether or not it was appropriate, so that if not, corrective action can be taken. And corrective action must not be punitive.

TP: Does someone else do the retroactive review or is it a self-reflection?

MM: Both.

TP: Marie, for 50 years, you've been living partnership in your personal life and your professional life. You've been a real visionary and pioneer in the field of Primary Nursing. And obviously Primary Nursing works. You've spoken internationally on this model, and many, many health care organizations use the Primary Nursing care delivery model. Can we discuss the cost of implementing the Primary Nursing model? Because people reading about this model for the first time might think, "Well, isn't that wonderful. But how can we possibly afford it?"

MM: The fact is that Primary Nursing does not cost any more money. It doesn't create any more work. I've never increased staffing in order to implement Primary Nursing.

TP: You've been talking about history repeating itself, and today we are seeing the same things: people not allowed to practice to the full extent of their education, hierarchical domination structures that oppress....

MM: We are still not stepping up to the plate. We need to be partnering with physicians. We need to be stepping into the interprofessional role.

TP: And to do that we need to have a strong sense of professional self-identity.

MM: We need to make the essence of nursing about relationships and not about functions.

TP: I believe the BASE of Nursing may help nurses discover their unique contribution. The BASE of Nursing shows that our relationship with clients, families, and communities is our unique medicine. It's so critical we understand that and bring that knowledge to the table.

MM: The roles that I'd really like to see nurses engaging in are partnering with patients; making sure that patients are participating in decision-making fully; and being advocates, making sure that the system is not harming the patient.

TP: So if a young person came to you today and said, "I'm thinking about being a nurse. Tell me three reasons why I should do that," what would you say?

MM: First of all, I'd say nursing is a privilege, a privilege that will expand the experience of your own life.

Two, it's a field that will facilitate and stimulate lifelong learning. There's nothing in the world that can't be brought into your awareness and your practice as a nurse. Whether it is astrophysics or geology—there is a truth, there is a relevance, to universal knowledge. Nursing gives you an opportunity to think as broadly as you possibly can.

And three, seeing what works in other people's lives, and what doesn't work, is a wonderful way of deciding how you're going to live your own life.

TP: Marie, it is such an honor to be with you today. I am in the presence of a living nursing legend. I appreciate the contribution you have made and continue to make to the profession of nursing, and I hope that your words help nurses to reclaim their power, their potential, and their partnership.

Marie Manthey used principles of partnership to develop a very effective and sustainable care delivery model. The model is based not only on respectful relationships with the patients but healthy relationships between nurses. The following sidebar offers all nurses a daily reminder to choose partnership over domination.

COMMITMENT TO MY COWORKERS FOR HEALTH CARE TEAMS

As your coworker, and with our shared organizational goal of excellent patient care, I commit to the following:

1. *I will accept responsibility for establishing and maintaining healthy interpersonal relationships with you and every other member of this team.*

2. *I will talk to you promptly if I am having a problem with you. The only time I will discuss it with another person is when I need advice or help in deciding how to communicate with you appropriately.*

3. *I will establish and maintain a relationship of functional trust with you and every member of this team. My relationships with each of you will be equally respectful, regardless of job title, level of education preparation, or any other differences that may exist.*

4. *I will not engage in the 3Bs (bickering, back-biting, and blaming). I will practice the 3Cs (caring, commitment, and collaboration) in my relationship with you and ask you to do the same with me.*

5. *I will not complain about another team member and ask you not to as well. If I hear you doing so, I will ask you to talk to that person.*

6. *I will accept you as you are today, forgiving past problems, and ask you to do the same with me.*

7. *I will be committed to finding solutions to problems, rather than complaining about them or blaming someone for them, and ask you to do the same.*

8. *I will affirm your contribution to the quality of our work.*

9. *I will remember that neither of us is perfect, and that human errors are opportunities not for shame or guilt, but for forgiveness and growth.*

Conclusion

Environments that decrease nursing unity and foster lateral violence effectively support domination values and agendas. Nurses need to realize that turning their anger and frustration at the system or toward one another does not change the system. Only partnership values and intraprofessional support can create healthy systems that engage employees and improve patient outcomes. Lateral violence is our greatest threat—working together as partners for change is our greatest hope.

References

American Academy of Nursing (AAN). (2013). Raise the voice. Retrieved from http://www.aannet.org/edgerunners

American Nurses Association (ANA). (2011). Lateral violence and bullying in nursing: Fact sheet. Retrieved from http://www.nursingworld.org/Mobile/Nursing-Factsheets/lateral-violence-and-bullying-in-nursing.html

Bartholomew, K. (2006). *Ending nurse-to-nurse hostility: Why nurses eat their young and each other.* Marblehead, MA: HCPro.

Caring Economy Campaign. (2011). The caring economy leadership program. Retrieved from http://www.caringeconomy.org/content/caring-economy-leadership-program

Center for Partnership Studies. (n.d.). Home page. Retrieved from http://www.partnershipway.org/

Daiski, I. (2004). Changing nurses' dis-empowering relationship patterns. *Journal of Advanced Nursing, 48*(1), 43-50.

Eisler, R. (n.d.). Shifting our relationships from domination to partnership. Retrieved from http://www.partnershipway.org/core-pathways/abcs-of-dominator-and-partnership-relations/copy_of_partnership-relationships

Eisler, R. (2000). *Tomorrow's children: A blueprint for partnership education in the 21ˢᵗ century.* Cambridge, MA: Westview Press.

Embree, J. L., & White, A. H. (2010). Concept analysis. Nurse-to-nurse lateral violence. *Nursing Forum, 45*(3), 166-173.

Freire, P. (1993). *Pedagogy of the oppressed* (Rev. ed.). New York: Continuum.

Institute for Safe Medication Practices (ISMP). (2004). Intimidation: Practitioners speak up about this unresolved problem. Retrieved from http://www.ismp.org/Newsletters/acutecare/articles/20040311_2.asp

Leape, L., Berwick, D., Clancy, C., Conway, J., Gluck, P., Guest, J.,...Isaac, T. (2009). Transforming healthcare: A safety imperative. *Quality Safety Health Care, 18*, 424-428. doi: 10.1136/qshc.2009.036954

Person, C. (2004). Patient care delivery. In M. Koloroutis (Ed.), *Relationship-based care: A model for transforming practice* (pp. 159-182). Minneapolis, MN: Creative Health Care Management.

Potter, T. M. (2010). Reconstructing a new story of nursing: Critical analysis of nursing textbooks using Riane Eisler's partnership paradigm. *Dissertation Abstracts International, 72*(05), 3447086.

Potter, T. M. (2013). *The BASE of nursing*. Unpublished manuscript, School of Nursing, University of Minnesota, United States of America.

Roberts, S. J. (1983). Oppressed group behavior: Implications for nursing. *Advances in Nursing Science, 5*(4), 21-30.

Roberts, S. J. (2000). Development of a positive professional identity: Liberating oneself from the oppressor within. *Advances in Nursing Science, 22*(4), 71-82.

Roberts, S. J., Demarco, R., & Griffin, M. (2009). The effect of oppressed group behaviors on the culture of the nursing workplace: A review of the evidence and interventions for change. *Journal of Nursing Management, 17*(3), 288-293.

Rowe, M. M., & Sherlock, H. (2005). Stress and verbal abuse: Do burned out nurses eat their young? *Journal of Nursing Management, 13*(3), 242-248.

Chapter 10
Partnership-Based
Interprofessional Relationships

*"Professionals have to work as partners in education and service
sectors equally sharing the responsibility for solving the major
practice-education gap."*

—Patricia Benner, PhD, RN (2012)

The growing interprofessional practice (IPP) movement is a major step forward, bringing together the knowledge and skills of professional teams to deliver health care more effectively. However, this movement must become anchored in partnership or it is doomed to failure or condemned to deliver the same ineffective outcomes.

This quote from a World Health Organization (WHO) document (2010) bears repeating because it makes this point so forcefully:

*Many health workers believe themselves to be practicing
collaboratively, simply because they work together with other
health workers ....Collaboration, however, is not only about
agreement and communication, but about creation and synergy.*

Collaboration occurs when two or more individuals from different backgrounds with complementary skills interact to create a shared understanding that none had previously possessed or could have come to on their own. (p. 36)

In other words, through a synergy grounded in a common goal and shared understanding, partnership brings results that go beyond individual contributions.

Identifying Patterns of Domination

Before going on to discuss partnership-based IPP models, we first need to identify some entrenched patterns of domination that stand in the way of effective interprofessional practice.

Advanced Nursing Practice

In 1860, Florence Nightingale established the first Nightingale Training School for nurses at St. Thomas' Hospital (Florence Nightingale Museum, n.d.). For the next 50 years, nursing education occurred exclusively within a hospital setting. In these hospital-based programs, nursing students earned certificates or diplomas in nursing in exchange for free labor. In 1909, visionary leaders at the University of Minnesota created the first School of Nursing within a university setting (University of Minnesota, 2013, "School of Nursing history" section). Nurses earned baccalaureate degrees comparable to other professions. Professional nursing later added graduate degree options, including the Master of Science in Nursing (MS or MSN), the Doctor of Philosophy (PhD), the Doctor of Science (DNS or DNSc), and the Doctor of Nursing Practice (DNP).

As a point of clarity, all nurses with advanced degrees are practicing in advanced nursing practice, but only some nurses with advanced degrees are advanced practice registered nurses.

Advanced practice registered nurses (APRNs) include nurse midwives, nurse anesthetists, clinical nurse specialists, and nurse practitioners. Originally, a master's degree was the required entrance degree for advanced practice nursing. However, in 2004, the American Association of Colleges of Nursing (AACN) issued a position paper stating that by 2015, the doctoral degree should be the entry-level degree for advanced practice nursing (AACN, 2004).

Several issues in health care prompted the AACN (2004) to take this position:

- Rapid expansion of knowledge required to function in interdisciplinary teams

- Increasing complexity of the health care system

- Concerns about the delivery of safe, cost-effective health care

- Demands for nurses to function at higher levels and help design systems that provide safe, cost-effective care

- Shortage of faculty required to prepare future nurses and leaders

- Specialist preparation programs that call for more credit hours than most graduate degrees require (Patzek, 2010, p. 49)

In short, the AACN concluded that a master's degree was no longer able to adequately prepare advanced practice nurses in light of these complex health care issues.

At that time, the nursing profession already had the PhD and the DNSc (or equivalent), with their strong emphasis on nursing research, but the profession was concerned that current issues in health care made it necessary for nurses to also have a practice doctorate option. This recognized need for a practice doctorate led to the creation of the Doctor of Nursing Practice (DNP), a degree comparable to the practice doctorates of other professions, including medicine (MD), law (JD), dentistry (DDS), pharmacy (PharmD), and physical therapy (DPT). To earn a DNP, students must obtain competencies in both a specialty area and advanced nursing practice in general. General competencies for the DNP are described in *The Essentials for Doctoral Education for Advanced Nursing Practice* (AACN, 2006).

The PhD, DNSc, and DNP all represent the highest academic degree in nursing. The research doctorates' (PhD or DNSc) focus is on the development of original knowledge. By contrast, the focus of the practice doctorate (DNP) is on translation of knowledge into practice. For example, nurse navigators are an emerging field in nursing. Their role is to assist patients and families to "navigate" the complex health care system. "Navigators help patients make informed medical decisions and assist with setting up multiple doctors' appointments and tests...make sure patients stay on track with their treatment plan and offer emotional support" (Landro, 2011). So, a PhD-prepared nurse might study this question: What is the impact on patient satisfaction scores when a *nurse navigator* is part of the interprofessional team? On the other hand the DNP-prepared nurse executive leader might use scientific literature to determine the most beneficial and cost-effective way to use nurse navigators in their hospital system.

Similar to Taoist philosophy where apparent opposites, Yin and Yang, are interconnected and interdependent, the PhD and DNP are likewise interdependent. New knowledge has minimal impact if it fails to find its way into practice, whereas practice that fails to be anchored in the most recent best evidence may fail to reach optimal outcomes for patients and communities. This, too, constitutes a kind of partnership. While some advanced nursing practice scholars (PhDs, DNSs) generate new knowledge, other advanced nursing practice scholars (DNPs) take that knowledge and translate the science into best practice. Neither of these paths to knowledge dominates; both influence and empower each other.

Yet patterns of domination, such as the ranking of one profession or degree over another, do persist within both intraprofessional and interprofessional practice. Meleis and Dracup (2005), two members of the nursing faculty from the University of Pennsylvania, describe a disturbing example of professional rankism within the academy. They write:

In most U.S. universities, membership in the academic Senate is granted to faculty members who hold tenured professorial ranks with the requirement of a PhD. Many DNP-prepared faculty will be excluded from the 'Senate' of universities, and thus will be excluded from having a voice and a vote in decision making pertaining to educational and faculty policies. Faculty members with the DNP, getting neither tenured positions nor Senate membership, will be barred from dialogues and discussions pertaining to their educational role. ("Marginalization" section)

Thus, the DNP, nursing's practice doctorate, and those who hold it, are marginalized due to an academic and professional hierarchy that denies these faculty members both tenure and a voice in decisions and policies.

Nurses need to know how to effectively respond to such ways of maintaining hierarchies of domination and other challenges that threaten the advancement of both nurses and nursing clinical knowledge.

Advanced Practice Registered Nurses (APRNs)

Several issues are currently prompting intense dialogue among providers, health care system executives, government agencies, patient advocacy groups, and others about who is qualified to provide primary care. These issues include health care reform, the call for patient-centered care, the need for teams of providers to deliver complex care, and the severe shortage of primary care providers. The United States is redefining the way primary care is delivered, and this can feel threatening to those still playing dominant roles.

The Institute of Medicine (IOM) report *The Future of Nursing: Leading Change, Advancing Health* (2010) recommends, "Nurses should practice to the full extent of their education and training" (p. S3). Yet nowhere is the limitation of practice more evident than with advanced practice registered nurses (APRNs). This is explicitly brought out in the IOM report, which states the following:

What nurse practitioners are able to do once they graduate varies widely for reasons that are related not to their ability, education or training, or safety concerns, but to the political decisions of the state in which they work. Depending on the state, restrictions on the scope of practice of an advanced practice registered nurse may limit or deny altogether the authority to prescribe medications, admit patients to the hospital, assess patient conditions, and order and evaluate tests. (p. S4)

It defies logic and a commitment to best practice to rule that nurse practitioners are not capable of being primary care providers when in another state nurses with the same degree practice autonomously.

At this time only 18 states and the District of Columbia allow nurse practitioners to diagnose, treat, and prescribe without physician supervision (Robert Wood Johnson Foundation [RWJF], 2013a), while in other states APRNs require supervision during activities such as diagnosing and prescribing medications. This rigid hierarchy between highly educated health care providers can negatively impact the quality and cost-effectiveness of health care.

STATES IN 2012 THAT ALLOWED NURSE PRACTITIONERS TO DIAGNOSE, TREAT, AND PRESCRIBE WITHOUT PHYSICIAN SUPERVISION (RWJF, 2013A)

Maine	*Vermont*	*New Hampshire*
Rhode Island	*Washington D.C.*	*Maryland*
New Mexico	*Arizona*	*Utah*
Colorado	*Hawaii*	*Washington*
Oregon	*Montana*	*Arkansas*
Idaho	*Wyoming*	*North Dakota*
Iowa		

Even where there are no formal rules discriminating against the nursing profession, patterns of subjugation and domination are very evident between some physicians and nurses. As a result, the relationship between physicians and APRNs is strained and contentious in many states. For example, referring to doctorally prepared APRNs, Harris (2011) reports for *The New York Times*:

Dr. Roland Goertz, the board chairman of the American Academy of Family Physicians, says that physicians are worried that losing control over 'doctor,' a word that has defined their profession for centuries, will be followed by the loss of control over the profession itself. He said that patients could be confused about the roles of various health professionals who all call themselves doctors. (para. 6)

This debate over who has the right to be called *doctor* is no trivial matter. Several state legislatures are pushing bills to limit use of the word *doctor* to physicians. For example, "a bill proposed in the New York State Senate would bar nurses from advertising themselves as doctors, no matter their degree" (Harris, 2011, para. 7). Control of the title *doctor* demonstrates that patterns of domination and subjugation continue to persist in interprofessional practice.

Another example of the efforts of physicians' associations to retain control is the following statement from "Primary Care for the 21st Century" (American Academy of Family Physicians, 2012):

Physicians offer an unmatched service to patients and without their skills patients would receive second-tier care. We must not downgrade Americans' care by offering them nurses instead of doctors. We can fill the need by having all health professionals on the team in the right roles. (p. 17)

Words like *second-tier* and *downgrade* clearly signal that the writers of the "Primary Care" article consider nursing an inferior profession. Indeed, this kind of thinking is still far too prevalent—even though research findings do not support the ranking of physicians over nurses in primary health care delivery.

Already over a decade ago, the question was raised about the difference between physician primary care providers and nurse primary care providers related to patient satisfaction and quality care outcomes. At that time Mundinger et al. (2000) conducted a randomized trial involving 1,316 patients from primary care clinics in the United States. A 6-month follow-up survey about satisfaction and health status, combined with a 1-year service utilization audit, showed that "patient outcomes for nurse practitioner and physician delivery of primary care do not differ" (p. 68).

Likewise, in the United Kingdom, Horrocks, Anderson, and Salisbury (2002) conducted research to determine whether nurses and physicians provide equivalent "first point of contact" primary care. The study reviewed randomized controlled studies and prospective observational studies. Findings indicated that patients overall were actually *more* satisfied with care provided by nurse practitioners. Moreover, there were no indications of differences in patient health status. The study also found that nurses spent longer time with patients and made more investigations than the physicians. The study concluded, "Nurse practitioners can provide care that leads to increased patient satisfaction and similar health outcomes when compared with care from a doctor. Nurse practitioners seemed to provide a quality of care that is at least as good, and in some ways better, than doctors" (Horrocks, Anderson, & Salisbury, 2002, p. 821).

The Cochrane Library, as previously mentioned, disseminates exhaustive reviews of current studies with the goal of setting the standard for evidence-based practice. Their review, "Substitution of Doctors by Nurses in Primary Care" (Laurant et al., 2004), found that when nurses are appropriately educated, the quality of their care as well as the patient health outcomes are equal to the care provided by primary care physicians.

Yet despite the Cochrane review's customary gold standard status, the American Academy of Family Physicians (AAFP) claimed the results of "Substitution of Doctors by Nurses in Primary Care" could not be generalized (Lindbloom, 2011). And Lindbloom (2011) reiterated the AAFP's assertion that nurse practitioners should not be independent primary care providers but instead only be part of an integrated practice team *under* the guidance of a physician. In these and other ways, the AAFP still takes a domination position rather than a partnership position related to interprofessional practice.

This continued derogation and subjugation of APRNs is sadly reminiscent of a 1901 issue of the *Journal of the American Medical Association* where some doctors claimed, "A nurse was often conceited and too unconscious of the due subordination she owes to the medical profession, of which she is sort of a useful parasite" (Walsh, as cited in Achterberg, 1990, p. 162). Continued domination and control of APRNs indicate we still have much work to do to manifest full partnership-based collaborative practice.

The good news is that some progress is being made. For example, in regard to who is qualified to provide primary care, the Robert Wood Johnson Foundation (RWJF, 2013a), an important stakeholder in the field of health care, summarized research findings as follows in their health policy brief "Nurse Practitioners and Primary Care":

> *The patient-centered nature of nurse practitioner training, which often includes care coordination and sensitivity to the impact on health of social and cultural factors, such as environment and family situation, makes nurse practitioners particularly well prepared for and interested in providing primary care. (p. 2)*

Furthermore, in "How to Fully Utilize the Skills, Knowledge, and Experience of Advanced Practice Registered Nurses," the RWJF (2013b) identifies and criticizes current legal, institutional, and cultural barriers that limit the full potential of APRNs. This policy brief also reports that interprofessional collaborative care may play a significant role in eliminating these barriers.

The time is ripe for a partnership-based model of interprofessional practice.

Partnership-Based Interprofessional Practice

Many experts are calling for interprofessional collaboration in light of the health care system's complexity (Bainbridge, Nasmith, Orchard, & Wood, 2010). This complexity requires a systems approach where problems are examined for the way they impact the entire organization, not just one part of the whole. For a systems approach to be effective, it requires a partnership perspective rather than a domination perspective (Eisler and Montuori, 2001).

This section looks at a systems approach developed by four prominent interprofessional education and collaborative practice (IPECP) scholars and at how it can be enriched and strengthened by using the partnership perspective.

IPECP scholars Bainbridge, Nasmith, Orchard, and Wood (2010) describe a systems approach to interprofessional competencies that include six interconnected domains:

- Role clarification

- Patient/client/family/community-centered care

- Team functioning

- Collaborative leadership

- Interprofessional communication

- Dealing with interprofessional conflict

Role Clarification

Competency Statement: Learners/practitioners understand their own role and the roles of those in other professions, and use this knowledge appropriately to establish and meet patient/client/family and community goals. (Bainbridge et al., 2010, p. 8)

As previously mentioned, the BASE of Nursing (Potter, 2013) is designed to give nurses increased clarity about their professional self-identity. Once nurses know who they are, it is easier to define and maintain boundaries about their role and the role of others.

In partnership models, if two or more professions have overlapping knowledge and skills, division of labor is respectfully negotiated. In the partnership paradigm, there can be a sense of trust and respect for interprofessional colleagues and a steadfast commitment to being allies for quality and cost-effective patient care.

Patient/Client/Family/Community-Centered Care

Competency Statement: Learners/practitioners seek out, integrate, and value, as a partner, the input, and the engagement of patient/client/family/community in designing and implementing care/services. (Bainbridge et al., 2010, p. 9)

This competency statement explicitly acknowledges the importance of real partnership, not just collaboration. Yet upon critical analysis of nursing fundamentals textbook content, Potter (2010) found that although the textbooks were in consensus about the importance of collaboration in health care, none of the textbooks explained how to create and maintain partnership in collaborative relationships.

Because our society still tends to embrace the domination perspective, this knowledge needs to be part of nursing education. We need to learn how to "seek out, integrate, and value as a partner" patients and communities. As described in previous chapters, Eisler's works (1987, 2002) are critical because they provide a template for partnership-based relationships, a requirement for effective interprofessional practice.

Team Functioning

Competency Statement: Learners/practitioners understand the principles of team dynamics and group processes to enable effective interprofessional team collaboration. (Bainbridge et al., 2010, p. 9)

Potter (2010) found in her research that throughout the history of nursing there has been recognition of the importance of partnership. For example, Dock and Stewart (1937), two early nurse historians, wrote the following:

If each group is to put forth its utmost effort, it must have a normal outlet for its intelligence and initiative as well as for its spirit of service. The arbitrary domination of one group by another is demoralizing to both and does not secure the best service of either. It is equally disastrous, however, for any one group to attempt to be completely independent and self-sufficient. Only by respecting the expert in his or her own field, and recognizing frankly the limitations of each group, shall we be able to work together harmoniously and effectively, and each take his full share in the common task. (p. 345)

When we recall and nurture nursing's historic commitment to the partnership perspective, we foster group dynamics that promote effective interprofessional teams. If at all possible, a partnership-based interprofessional practice avoids hierarchies. In situations where they are required, the IPECP participants practice *hierarchies of actualization*, where the team leader or manager inspires, facilitates, and guides rather than controls the group (Eisler, 2002).

Collaborative Leadership

Competency Statement: Learners/practitioners understand and can apply leadership principles that support a collaborative practice model. (Bainbridge et al., 2010, p. 9)

Too often a physician assumes leadership of an interprofessional team without the input of the other professions on the team. In these situations, if a physician is on the team, that physician assumes she or he will lead.

In partnership models, however, when collaboration requires leadership, the leader is selected based on the skill set required by the team's particular needs, rather than on the basis of professional hierarchies. Any team member potentially can lead the group.

Eisler and Montuori (2001) write, "In partnership systems, the orientation to 'power to' or actualizing power and 'power-with' leads to a very different attitude, one that starts off by asking, 'how can we best work together to solve problems?'" (p. 13). Leadership based on principles of partnership creates an environment where effective collaborative teams can thrive.

Interprofessional Communication

Competency Statement: Learners/practitioners from varying professions communicate with each other in a collaborative, responsive, and responsible manner. (Bainbridge et al., 2010, p. 9)

Fear obscures facts and limits innovation—and domination systems tend to engender fear. If we want to develop novel solutions to complex health issues, we must create safe environments where respectful communication is the norm. In partnership organizations, opinions and observations can be shared without fear. In the partnership paradigm, no one feels the need to control or limit a colleague. Therefore, communication can be more thoughtful, open, and respectful.

Dealing with Interprofessional Conflict

Competency Statement: Learners/practitioners actively engage self and others, including the client/patient/family, in positively and constructively addressing interprofessional conflict as it arises. (Bainbridge et al., 2010, p. 9)

Conflict between different perspectives is not the problem; the problem is how conflict is handled. In partnership-based interprofessional practice, participants use civil conversation and respectful behavior to resolve disagreements. Violence and abuse, both physical and verbal, are not tolerated.

Conflicts also arise in partnership relationships, but how these are handled is very different from how conflict is handled in the domination paradigm, where conflict is used to win at all costs. In the context of partnership, "conflict is creatively used to arrive at solutions (Eisler, n.d., "Myths about Partnership"). Of course, some conflicts cannot be resolved in either context. But in a partnership system, conflict can be an opportunity to learn, communicate, and craft innovative solutions.

Partnership Exemplar: Nurse-Managed Health Centers

The nursing story continues. Following in the footsteps of Lillian Wald, Margaret Sanger, Mary Breckinridge, and Sister Elizabeth Kenny, nurses today continue creating new models of care delivery in response to emerging and unmet needs. Nurse-managed health centers (NMHCs) integrate health promotion, disease prevention, and primary care, and deliver it where it is needed most: in underserved, vulnerable communities.

NMHCs can be found in rural and urban churches, synagogues and mosques, schools, Native American reservations, homeless shelters, and even shopping malls. The centers are generally staffed with transdisciplinary or interprofessional teams of nurse practitioners, clinical nurse specialists, social workers, behavioral health specialists, psychologists, midwives, public health nurses, community outreach workers, academic faculty, health care students, and physicians (National Nursing Centers Consortium, 2011).

The underlying principle of nurse-managed health care centers is partnership. The National Nursing Centers Consortium (2011) states:

> We know our patients and our patients know and trust us. We take the time to listen and to learn about the whole person, and consequently make the connections between a person's life and the state of his or her health. ("Nurse-Managed Health Centers Today section)

NMHCs manifest the BASE of Nursing (Potter, 2013), including commitment to presence and using the unique stories of individuals and the community to guide practice.

11th Street Family Health Services, Drexel University

An example of a nurse-managed health center is 11th Street Family Health Services. Like other NMHCs, the goal of 11th Street Family Health Services is to:

Work in partnership with the community to develop a healthy living center that is community-based and culturally relevant, providing not only access to clinical services but also a wide range of health promotion and disease prevention services to reduce health disparities in an underserved population. (American Academy of Nursing, 2012)

This partnership between professionals and other health disciplines creates an environment where synergy thrives and effective approaches to health are implemented.

Dr. Patricia Garrity, associate dean for community programs at Drexel University, writes of the partnership-based relationship between professionals in the 11th Street model as *transdisciplinary*. She states, "Transdisciplinary means you start to break down the barriers between disciplines. Each person learns something about the other person's discipline, and it enriches their own practice" (Initiative on the Future of Nursing, 2011). Typically patients must attend one clinic for their physical health care needs and another clinic for their mental health needs, but at the 11th Street Family Health Services, behavioral health and primary health care are seamlessly integrated.

This collaboration of behavioral health and primary care strengthens the services provided to patients by placing a primary behavioral health specialist and social worker directly in primary care. The primary behavioral health therapist focuses on the patient's mental health, and the social worker addresses any social service needs and linkages (Innovative Care Models, 2008).

In addition to behavioral health and primary care, 11th Street Family Health Services also provide a wide range of other health services including dental services, physical therapy, family planning, nutrition counseling, and social work.

True to the partnership model, 11th Street Family Health Services also empowers clients, young and old, to be full partners in their own health. To do this, the organization offers targeted programs and services, including "Teens 4 Good Urban Farming," "Chronic Disease Self Management," and a fitness center with a fitness trainer (Drexel University College of Nursing and Health Professions, 2010a, Services & Programs).

The *Guiding Principles of 11th Street Family Health Services* reflect a deep commitment to a partnership paradigm:

- We put the patient first and follow a model of care that uses our resources wisely to provide for the needs of our patients, our staff, and our community.

- We work in partnership with the community and the university to improve the health status of the community.

- We provide services based on community-defined needs.

- We provide access to high-quality health care for all, regardless of their ability to pay.

- We collaborate and communicate with the utmost integrity to support an environment of trust and respect among our patients/clients, staff, and community.

- We are dedicated, enthusiastic, highly skilled staff committed to providing care and service. We value diversity, respect the dignity of all, and accept the uniqueness of individuals.

- We promote innovation and a willingness to try new approaches with vitality, energy, and enthusiasm in order to support change and foster growth (Drexel University College of Nursing and Health Professions, 2010b, Facts and Figures).

In reviewing these principles, you can clearly discern partnership themes—respect, diversity, safe, two-way communication, innovation, and *hierarchies of actualization*. As described in previous chapters, a partnership approach not only creates a positive work environment, but it also directly improves health outcomes and markedly decreases health disparities. For example, the 11th Street Family Health Services:

- Reduced pre-term births to 2.5% in African American women seen at 11th Street compared to 15.6% in Philadelphia.

- Improved quality of life for patients participating in the fitness program, as measured by the SF 36, a short-form health survey with 36 questions measuring health and well-being. There was a significant increase in perceived health status at 3-, 6-, and 12-month followups.

- Decreased unnecessary medical specialty workups for children whose issues (such as enuresis) are family/behaviorally based through the integration of a pediatric behavioral health consultant in primary care (American Academy of Nursing, 2012, "Evidence of Success").

Not surprisingly, the 11th Street Family Health Services:

- Received a Healthy Workplace Award from the *Philadelphia Business Journal* for its efforts to provide time and opportunities for staff to participate in health-promoting activities.

- Was included as a case study in the IOM (2010) report *The Future of Nursing* to illustrate that community partnerships reduce health disparities.

- Was named on the Innovation Exchange of the federal Agency for Health Quality Research (AHQR) for opening access to care (American Academy of Nursing, 2012, "Evidence of Success").

These results are not unique to 11th Street Family Health Services. Nurse-managed clinics around Philadelphia are seeing similar results from a partnership-based interprofessional approach. For example, a significant finding about the positive features of these clinics is that nurses "see their patients almost twice as often as other providers; their patients are hospitalized 30% less and use the emergency room 15% less often than those of other health care providers" (National Nursing Centers Consortium, 2011).

Clearly, nursing and nurse-managed clinics offer excellent returns on investment and are a very exciting model for interprofessional collaborative practice.

Conclusion

Hierarchies of domination are the single greatest threat to effective interprofessional practice. Adopting a partnership perspective will ensure that professionals practice to the full extent of their education, that communication flows freely and different views and insights are respected. In partnership-based interprofessional practice the emphasis is on the needs of patients and families instead of one professional's need to control others.

References

Achterberg, J. (1990). *Woman as healer*. Boston, MA: Shambhala.

American Academy of Family Physicians (AAFP). (2012). Primary care for the 21ˢᵗ century: Ensuring a quality physician-led team for every patient. Retrieved from http://www.aafp.org/online/en/home/membership/initiatives/nps/patientcare.html

American Academy of Nursing (AAN). (2012). Raise the voice edge runner: 11th Street Family Health Services, Drexel University. Retrieved from http://www.aannet.org/assets/docs/RaisetheVoice/EdgeRunnerProfiles/2012NewProfiles/rtv_11th%20street%20family%20health%20services_web.pdf

American Association of Colleges of Nursing (AACN). (2004). AACN position statement on the practice doctorate in nursing. Retrieved from http://www.aacn.nche.edu/dnp/faqs

American Association of Colleges of Nursing (AACN). (2006). The essentials for doctoral education for advanced nursing practice. Retrieved from http://www.aacn.nche.edu/education-resources/essential-series

Bainbridge, L., Nasmith, L., Orchard, C., & Wood, V. (2010). Competencies for interprofessional collaboration. *Journal of Physical Therapy Education, 24*(1), 6-11.

Benner, P. (2012). Urgently needed: A radical transformation of professional collaboration and teamwork. Retrieved from http://www.educatingnurses.com/articles/interprofessional-education/

Dock, L. L., & Stewart, I. M. (1937). *A short history of nursing: From the earliest times to the present day* (3rd ed., rev.). New York: G. P. Putnam's Sons.

Drexel University College of Nursing and Health Professions. (2010a). 11th Street Family Health Services: Services and programs. Retrieved from http://www.drexel.edu/11thstreet/services.asp

Drexel University College of Nursing and Health Professions. (2010b). Facts and figures about 11th Street Family Health Services of Drexel University. Retrieved from http://www.drexel.edu/11thstreet/facts.asp

Eisler, R. (n.d.). Myths about partnership. Retrieved from http://www.partnershipway.org/core-pathways/abcs-of-dominator-and-partnership-relations/two-social-possibilities-the-domination-system-and-the-partnership-system/?searchterm=conflict

Eisler, R. (1987). *The chalice and the blade: Our history, our future.* San Francisco, CA: Harper & Row.

Eisler, R. (2002). *The power of partnership: Seven relationships that will change your life.* Novato, CA: New World Library.

Eisler, R., & Montuori, A. (2001). The partnership organization a systems approach. *OD Practitioner, 33*(2), 11-17.

Florence Nightingale Museum. (n.d.). Florence's biography. Retrieved from http://www.florence-nightingale.co.uk/the-collection/biography.html

Harris, G. (2011, October 1). When the nurses wants to be called doctor. *The New York Times.* Retrieved from http://www.nytimes.com/2011/10/02/health/policy/02docs.html?pagewanted=all&_r=0

Horrocks, S., Anderson, E., & Salisbury, C. (2002). Systematic review of whether nurse practitioners working in primary care can provide equivalent care to doctors. *BMJ, 324,* 819-823.

Initiative on the Future of Nursing. (2011). Eleventh Street Family Health Services of Drexel University. Retrieved from http://thefutureofnursing.org/resource/detail/eleventh-street-family-health-services-drexel-university

Innovative Care Models. (2008). 11th Street Family Health Services. Retrieved from http://www.innovativecaremodels.com/care_models/16/key_elements

Institute of Medicine (IOM). (2010). *The future of nursing: Leading change, advancing health.* Washington, DC: National Academies Press.

Landro, L. (2011, August 16). When a doctor isn't enough: Nurse navigators help patients through maze of cancer-treatment decisions, fears. *The Wall Street Journal.* Retrieved from http://online.wsj.com/article/SB1000142405311190425320457651047282828240848.html

Laurant, M., Reeves, D., Hermens, R., Braspenning, J., Grol, R., & Sibbald, B. (2004). Substitution of doctors by nurses in primary care. *Cochrane Database of Systematic Reviews, 4,* (CD001271).

Lindbloom, E. (2011). Evidence substituting nurses for primary care physicians is lacking. *AAFP*. Retrieved from http://www.aafp.org/online/en/home/publications/news/news-now/opinion/20111123npeditorial.html

Meleis, A. I., & Dracup, K. (2005). The case against the DNP: History, timing, substance, and marginalization. *Online Journal of Issues in Nursing, 10*(3), (8p), (13 ref).

Mundinger, M. O., Kane, R. L., Lenz, E. R., Totten, A. M., Tsai, W. Y., Cleary, P. D.,...Shelanski, M. L. (2000). Primary care outcomes in patients treated by nurse practitioners or physicians: A randomized trial. *JAMA, 283*(1), 59-68.

National Nursing Centers Consortium. (2011). *About nurse-managed care.* Retrieved from http://www.nncc.us/site/index.php/about-nurse-managed-care

Patzek, M. J. (May, 2010). Understanding the DNP degree. *American Nurse Today, 5*(5), 49-50. Retrieved from http://www.americannursetoday.com/article.aspx?id=6656&fid=6592

Potter, T. M. (2010). Reconstructing a new story of nursing: Critical analysis of nursing textbooks using Riane Eisler's partnership paradigm. *Dissertation Abstracts International, 72*(05), 3447086.

Potter, T. M. (2013). *The BASE of nursing.* Unpublished manuscript, School of Nursing, University of Minnesota, United States of America.

Robert Wood Johnson Foundation (RWJF). (2013a). Health policy brief: Nurse practitioners and primary care. *Health Affairs, May 15, 2013.* Retrieved from http://www.rwjf.org/content/dam/farm/reports/issue_briefs/2013/rwjf402293

Robert Wood Johnson Foundation (RWJF). (2013b). How to fully utilize the skills, knowledge, and experience of advanced practice registered nurses. *Charting Nursing's Future, 20,* 1-8. Retrieved from http://www.rwjf.org/en/research-publications/find-rwjf-research/2009/01/charting-nursings-future-archives/improving-patient-access-to-high-quality-care.html

University of Minnesota. (2013). School of nursing history. Retrieved from http://www.nursing.umn.edu/about/history/index.htm

World Health Organization (WHO). (2010). *Framework for action on interprofessional education and collaborative practice.* WHO Department of Human Resources for Health. Geneva, Switzerland: WHO Press.

Chapter 11
Partnership With Communities

"Go to the people. Live with them. Learn from them. Love them. Start with what they know. Build with what they have. But with the best leaders, when the work is done, the task accomplished, the people will say, 'We have done this ourselves.'"

–Attributed to Lao Tzu

Public health is not a new idea. It can trace its roots back to the earliest indigenous healers whose aim was to maintain the mind/body/spirit health of the entire tribe in relation to the environment. Later, water and waste management were recognized as critical for the survival of early civilizations. The field of epidemiology began in 1854 when John Snow used scientific analysis to trace a London cholera outbreak to a polluted public well. His success illuminated the possibilities of science-based prevention.

In the middle of the last century, the arrival of antibiotics prompted a cultural swing from prevention to acute care. Simply put, why do we need to work so hard to prevent illness when a pill can solve the issue? Acute care rapidly became the dominant paradigm, and up until now most of the spotlight has been on new drugs, new surgical interventions, new medical devices, and lifesaving care.

Public and community health have continued to do remarkable prevention, health promotion, and chronic illness care, but this work has remained in the shadows of acute care.

The tide is changing, however. We have come to realize that when the acute care paradigm dominates, sustainability is not possible. We need to reprioritize the focus of health care, placing emphasis on primary prevention and healthy communities. But as you have seen in other chapters, it is not enough to reprioritize, because even public health and community health can be viewed and administered from a domination perspective. This chapter describes partnership-based community care and offers a very successful community model anchored in partnership principles.

DOMINATION-BASED COMMUNITY CARE

A community or public health program functioning from the domination paradigm would take the following approach.

Mission: *To make sure community members comply with approved public health initiatives outlined by the state legislature and the state department of health.*

Role of Health Care Workers: *The role of community health care workers is to prioritize the needs of individuals or groups, allocate scarce resources, implement best practice initiatives, and document outcomes.*

Measurement of Success: *Success will be measured by significant improvement of health outcomes during the assigned allocation period. Funding will not be renewed if the health outcome objectives have not been met.*

Threads of Domination:

- *Rigid hierarchies*
- *Top-down communication and planning*
- *Emphasis on scarcity rather than abundance*
- *Interventions based on knowledge only from science (evidence-based practice), excluding knowledge from the community*
- *Unrealistic time table for real and lasting change*
- *Threat of funding withdrawal promotes fear and uncertainty*

Historic Context of Community Care

The story of nursing (Chapters 4 and 5) reminds us that the earliest roots of nursing were in the community. Nurses provided autonomous care for a wide variety of patients and conditions. These early nurses applied bandages, administered herbal remedies, were midwives to women giving birth, comforted the dying, and taught the community about health and wellness.

In more recent times, Lillian Wald, a public health and school nursing visionary, actually went to the people and lived with them. She learned from them and built on what they knew. In partnership with the community, she empowered them to live healthier lives. Yet for most of modern history, community care and hospital care have remained in rigidly separated silos. This separation only began to change a few decades ago—and then primarily for financial rather than health care reasons.

In the early 1980s, in response to fears of looming Medicare insolvency, the United States government initiated the Prospective Payment System (PPS). This system involves the International Classification of Diseases (ICD), diagnostic-related groups (DRG), and reimbursement based on the expected cost of care for a particular disease rather than the cost of actual services provided (Mayes, 2007). In response to PPS, hospitals scrambled to establish hospital-based home care programs where subacute care could be delivered more cost effectively in the home while still keeping revenues within the hospital system.

This rapid expansion of services into the community led to care being delivered by many different providers, including public health or visiting nurse services, hospital-based home care and hospice programs, and for-profit home care services. Some of these programs provided a full scope of services for clients of different ages and conditions, whereas other programs were more specialized (for example, pediatric care, hospice care, or infusion therapy).

As acute care expanded into the community, the domination perspective reasserted its hold. The "business of health care" began to dominate community care. For instance, community nurses once acted autonomously, delivering all the care that people needed to stay in their own homes. Now Medicare only reimburses skilled care that has been ordered by a physician. Not only that, for Medicare coverage of nursing services at home, the client has to be medically homebound. In other words, Medicare covers care only when it is a severe hardship for clients to leave their home for medical treatment.

This model displays several threads of domination. First of all, community nurses and other professionals who are well versed in a home care client's situation and care needs find their presence controlled by physicians. That is, even if a client or family directly requests skilled services, the nurse can go out to the home only when ordered by a physician. Furthermore, even when the nurse obtains an order to go out to the home, she or he must obtain additional physician orders if she or he deems that social worker, home health aide, or dietitian visits are warranted. This professional hierarchy diminishes nurses' ability to effectively coordinate care. It creates gaps in care and prevents timely delivery of services. Pulling care-coordination skills away from the nurse also creates a system that requires more middle managers, resulting in increased overhead.

Also, in this model, Medicare reimburses services only if home care clients require skilled nursing care, such as assessment of a changing condition, patient education related to a new medication or medication change, the complex dressing change of a wound, or the administration of an injection or IV medication. The need for skilled care must also be part time or intermittent, which means that Medicare will not pay unless the needed nursing care requires fewer than 7 days each week, or fewer than 8 hours each day, over a period of 21 days (Centers for Medicare & Medicaid Services, n.d.). In other words, Medicare will *not* reimburse for ongoing or chronic care needs.

This model reflects a top-down paradigm in which people who may never actually *see* the client and family control the quality and quantity of nursing care. The client has very little opportunity to share responsibility, and the model still fails to focus on prevention, with negative outcomes for both patients and taxpayers. And this approach leaves almost no room for innovation or for other delivery models.

This is all in conformity with the domination rather than the partnership model. Even though care is delivered in the home, and clients and families often perform many of the interventions themselves, they still are not full partners in their own care. For the most part they are passive recipients of care "ordered" by someone else, rather than being informed participants in their own care design.

The economic drivers of this home care model force the nurse to stray far from nursing's earlier, more partnership-oriented roots, and it fails to offer the family-centered care that can effectively meet the client's needs.

Figure 11.1 illustrates the rising costs of health care over the years.

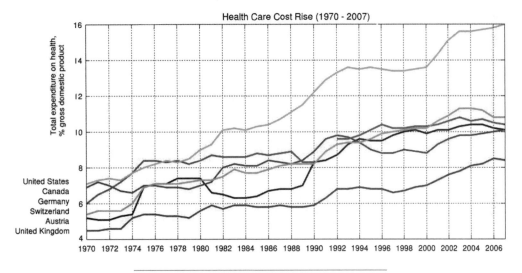

FIGURE 11.1 HEALTH CARE COST RISE.

Community Care Related to the Patient Protection and Affordable Care Act

On March 23, 2010, President Barack Obama signed the Patient Protection and Affordable Care Act (PPACA) into law. This sweeping piece of legislation, largely focused on insurance reform, proposes a new delivery model called *Accountable Care Organizations* (ACOs). The Centers for Medicare & Medicaid Services (CMS) states:

> *Accountable Care Organizations (ACOs) are groups of doctors, hospitals, and other health care providers, who come together voluntarily to give coordinated high quality care to their Medicare patients. The goal of coordinated care is to ensure that patients, especially the chronically ill, get the right care at the right time, while avoiding unnecessary duplication of services and preventing medical errors. (CMS, 2013, para. 1)*

The ACOs are designed to meet this *Triple Aim*: delivering quality care that satisfies client needs, improving the health of populations, and decreasing the per capita cost of health care (Institute for Healthcare Improvement [IHI], 2013, para. 1). ACOs also have the potential to move much closer to a partnership-based system of care.

Eisler (1987, 2002) reminds us that social systems are not all partnership or all domination, but rather move along a continuum from one pole to the other. Her macro-historical methodology also makes it possible to see the shifts between the domination and partnership perspectives, and that even after the shift to a domination orientation, there were still periods of movement toward the partnership side. Moreover, whether a society is primarily domination-based or partnership-based is not immutable. Eisler teaches us that we are not destined to live with a faulty system. Cultures are human creations, and we can build a system that works better for everyone.

While they may not use this language, many scholars have been pointing to the shortcomings of the old domination model of health care. Equally important is that we are beginning to see that we can create new, more sustainable, more effective, partnership-based models of care.

Partnership-Based Community Care

Designing partnership-based community nursing care requires three major ingredients:

- The first is a strong professional nursing identity based on our shared nursing story.

- The second is practice of the full BASE of Nursing medicine (Potter, 2013).

- The third is an effective partnership framework to guide the design of community care.

Eisler and Montuori (2001) outline this framework in "The Partnership Organization: A Systems Approach." Originally, the target audience for this article was organizational development practitioners (defined as those people "with the ultimate responsibility to develop and create organizational-wide effectiveness through challenging and changing its current practices") (Human Resource in a Nutshell, 2011). These days, nurses are frequently called to play this role in their health care organizations. Therefore Eisler and Montuori's framework is directly pertinent to the nursing profession.

Eisler and Montuori's (2001) framework for partnership organizations includes seven concepts:

- Flatter, less rigid hierarchical organizations

- Change in the role of the manager, from "the cop" to a facilitator, supportive role

- From "power over" to "power with" and "power to"

- Teamwork

- Diversity

- Gender balance

- Creativity and entrepreneurship (p. 12-14)

Each of these concepts needs to be intentionally addressed by all of us in order for partnership-based community care models to be effective.

Flatter, Less Rigid Hierarchical Organizations

Partnership-based community care models have more providers and fewer administrators. This is because each nurse will manage her or his own work assignments and maintain her or his own relationships with primary care providers, clinics, and hospitals. With fewer rigid hierarchies, partnership-based community care organizations are able to implement the Institute of Medicine's (IOM, 2010) recommendation that nurses practice to the full extent of their education. In addition, such models allow nurses to practice more holistically and cost effectively. In partnership-based models, care providers, clients, and families can work together to determine the most efficient way to deliver the necessary care.

COMMUNITY CARE: FLATTER, LESS RIGID HIERARCHICAL ORGANIZATIONS

Ideas and communication flow freely between all members of the community organization. Community representatives are involved in all aspects of community programming including conducting a needs assessment, grant writing, budget decisions, implementation of initiatives, and community education.

Change in the Role of the Manager From "Cop" to Facilitator

Partnership-based community care organizations implement *hierarchies of actualization* (Eisler, 2002) rather than hierarchies of domination. This enables nurses to use their power and influence to help others reach their full intellectual and creative potential.

Eisler and Montuori's (2001) model guides nurses to focus more on outcomes than micro-management. This shift in focus facilitates a "mutual learning loop" (p. 13) where nurses learn as well as teach, which is an optimal relationship for family-centered care in the community. Applying the BASE of Nursing (Potter, 2013), health care workers are present to the emerging and evolving needs of clients, families, and whole communities. Ongoing relationships based on trust allow stories and narratives to emerge. These narratives help guide the planning and implementation of client-, family-, and community-driven initiatives.

COMMUNITY CARE: CHANGE IN THE ROLE OF THE MANAGER, FROM "THE COP" TO A FACILITATOR

The leader of the community-based care initiative is selected based on expertise related to the initiative and ability to support and foster a partnership-based team. When a hierarchy is necessary, it takes the form of a hierarchy of actualization rather than a hierarchy of domination. The emphasis is always on engagement, inclusivity, and empowerment of those with less power.

From *Power Over* to *Power With* and *Power To*

In partnership-based community care, power is shared, and it is used to empower, rather than disempower, others. Eisler and Montuori (2001) state the following:

An important aspect of the partnership model is the reconceptualization of power from Power Over—the power to control and dominate others and our environment—to Power With and Power To; in other words, the capacity to work to achieve goals with others, but not at the expense of others. This is a shift from domination to co-creation, or from coercive power to generative power. (p. 13)

Instead of coming to the client with all the solutions, the nurse approaches the client with two key questions: What are your health care goals? How can we work together to help you reach your goals? This approach empowers clients to fully participate in improving their own health. In addition, once the services are no longer needed, the clients are confident in their own abilities and are not dependent on external experts to maintain their health.

COMMUNITY CARE: FROM "POWER OVER" TO "POWER WITH" AND "POWER TO"

When community members are included in planning community initiatives and in implementation of care, power is shared. As mentioned previously, power is shared with people and communities and given to communities to participate in solving their community's or family's self-defined needs.

Teamwork

Much is said these days about collaborative care. Yet collaboration is not the only requirement for effective teams. As Eisler and Montuori (2001) write, "If efforts at creating successful teams are not accompanied by a shift from a dominator to a partnership way of relating, most efforts will in fact be doomed" (p. 13).

As explained in Chapter 10, partnership-based teams are committed to a type of relationship that is significantly different from that of the conventional medical model. Not only are goals and objectives the focus, but healthy and mutually respectful relationships between team members are also paramount. When team members feel safe and experience mutual respect, synergy and innovation are possible, and new ideas and approaches develop.

Partnership-based community care teams span boundaries, bringing allies together to work on complex systems issues. Without hierarchies of domination, the need to control conversations and meetings decreases. In its place, the free and creative exchange of ideas makes the team more efficient at recognizing the highest quality, most cost-effective health care solutions.

> ### COMMUNITY CARE: TEAMWORK
>
> *Partnership-based community care recognizes that complex public health challenges will be solved only when the expertise of the community combines with the expertise of an interprofessional health care team.*

Diversity

From a dominator perspective, diversity is a threat. But from a partnership perspective, diversity is an opportunity for greater creativity, for sharing new perspectives, and creating new ideas and relationships. Diversity presents possibilities for unusual and generative cross-pollinations (Eisler & Montuori, 2001, p. 14).

Every year, *Fortune* magazine ranks the 500 companies that are most successful based on revenues. Many of these companies also make diversity a top priority. *Fortune* also compiles a list of the 50 best organizations for minorities. According to Chen, Harrington, Lustgarten, Mero, and Tkaczyk (2004), the 50 top firms "make an effort not only to hire minorities but also to retain them and promote them through the ranks. They actively interact with outside minority communities, and make management accountable for diversity efforts" (para. 4). Medical facilities and insurance and managed care companies regularly make the Fortune 500 list, but *not one* of these health care organizations made the list of the 50 best places for minority employees (Chen et al., 2004). There is a major diversity disconnect in health care.

According to United States Census Bureau (2012) projections, the United States will become a *majority-minority nation* in 2043. This means even though the non-Hispanic white population will remain the largest group, no group will make up a majority. Unless things radically change, the health care professions will continue to fail to mirror the people they serve. In a national sample survey of registered nurses conducted in 2008, 83% of U.S. registered nurses were white, while only 65% of the U.S. population was white. Minority nurses made up only 16.8% of all nurses (Health Resources and Services Administration [HRSA], 2010, section 7-5).

In a partnership-based community health care organization, the care providers and staff will not only more closely mirror the community they serve but ideally live within the community. As you read in the settlement movement initiated by Lillian Wald, significant advantages occur when health workers come from within the community.

This philosophy is reflected in a growing partnership-based health care delivery model known as the *community health worker* (CHW) initiative. In this delivery model, selected and respected members of a community are trained to care for their community by providing basic health and medical care. This "task shifting" strategy is part of the World Health Organization's (WHO, 2008) goal to make quality care available to all people despite the severe worldwide shortage of health care workers.

COMMUNITY CARE: DIVERSITY

In partnership-based community care, diversity is not only valued, but also essential for successful initiatives. Homogeneity in any form—gender, ethnicity, age, education, etc.—decreases the ability to discern the most optimal solutions.

Gender Balance

In most professions "gender balance" refers to making sure there are as many opportunities for women as there are for men. However, in nursing, the gender imbalance is flipped. In 2011, only 9% of all nurses were male (United States Census Bureau, 2013).

Yet even though the majority of nurses are female, old patterns of domination persist. The United States Census Bureau (2013) found that "women working as nurses full time, year-round earned 91 cents for every dollar male nurses earned" (para. 5). Not only that, a study of the experience of male nursing students found, "In clinical settings, male nursing students thought they were treated better by physicians than their female counterparts and were perceived as stable employees who would easily 'move up the ladder' in nursing" (MacWilliams, Schmidt, & Bleich, 2013, p. 41). In the same study, "male nursing students perceived that clinical instructors had different expectations of them than they had of their female peers—that they should be assertive, act as leaders, and take on lifting tasks—and female peers seemed to share these expectations" (p. 42). These examples represent the classic domination pattern of ranking males over females—a pattern that also accounts for the devaluation of the largely female nursing profession.

In comparison, Eisler and Montuori (2001) observed this in partnership organizations:

There is a holistic and synergistic view of identity. Individuals are not locked into restrictive, stereotypical gender roles, but free to express all their potential. They can experience and express feelings, thoughts and behaviors they deem appropriate, regardless of how they are gender-specifically categorized. While a fundamental characteristic of partnership systems is that they are gender-balanced and holistic, dominator systems polarize and accentuate socially and historically constructed gender differences. (p. 14)

Equally important, which you examine in Chapter 13, is that partnership-oriented organizations are conscious of what Eisler calls the *hidden system* of gendered valuations that devalues not only women but activities stereotypically associated with the "feminine"—along with active efforts to leave that distorted system of values behind.

A partnership-based community care organization will therefore strive for gender equity both in hiring practices and in salaries. Both male and female nurses will be expected to exhibit both critical thinking and caring expertise, and neither gender will be viewed as being more suitable for nursing than the other.

COMMUNITY CARE: GENDER BALANCE

Community care does not support old domination thinking that only women provide nurturing care and only men are analytical. Both genders are valued for their ability to manifest the full scope of comprehensive community care.

Creativity and Entrepreneurship

The complex interconnected system we call "community" may prove to be the most fruitful environment for partnership, since in many ways communities have often resisted giving themselves fully over to domination. As Eisler (1987, 2002) documents in her books, artists, designers, philosophers, activists, ecologists, and others throughout history have pulled community toward the partnership side of the continuum. As the story of nursing (Chapters 4 and 5) demonstrates, new models of family-centered care often get their start in the community.

More than ever, as we move to reform health care, we need to make space for creativity and new ways of thinking via social entrepreneurship. According to Ashoka, the largest worldwide social entrepreneur network:

> *Social entrepreneurs are individuals with innovative solutions to society's most pressing social problems. They are ambitious and persistent, tackling major social issues and offering new ideas for wide-scale change. Rather than leaving societal needs to the government or business sectors, social entrepreneurs find what is not working and solve the problem by changing the system, spreading the solution, and persuading entire societies to take new leaps. (Ashoka, n.d., "What is a Social Entrepreneur?")*

Social entrepreneurship is a wonderful example of partnership-based creativity. Eisler and Montuori (2001) write about creativity and explain its relationship to the domination/partnership continuum:

> *In dominator systems, there is an ambiguous relationship with creativity: it is viewed as a great gift, and at the same time potentially enormously disruptive, a threat to the established order. In partnership systems, creativity is both highly valued and rewarded. While partnership creativity does not exclude dramatic creative changes, it also fosters creative relationships and creative approaches to everyday problems. (p. 14)*

In other words, creativity is not considered the monopoly of a few exceptional people (mostly men, according to the conventional canon). What scholars today call *everyday creativity* is recognized and greatly valued—all the way from the "women's work" of creating a pleasing home environment and mothering to educational approaches that help children find their special gifts (rather than expecting each child to fit a predetermined mold as when "teaching to the test").

Similarly in a partnership-based health care system, creativity and novel thinking are not seen as a threat to health care students, faculty, or practitioners. In fact, this type of health care system does everything possible to nurture environments where innovation can thrive. In partnership-based community care, all the stakeholders are significant participants in creating the best system to serve the community. Just because "it has never been done" does not mean it cannot be done. Innovative thinking and problem solving are regular features of the system, as are flexibility and nimbleness. Instead of being imparted rigidly solidified knowledge, participants are taught how to learn and where to go for information. Care providers and care recipients partner to cocreate a sustainable quality system for all.

COMMUNITY CARE: CREATIVITY AND ENTREPRENEURSHIP

Again, old thinking and old processes will only continue to produce the same results. If we really want to reform the health care system in the United States, we need to be willing to think differently. In community care this may mean moving beyond traditional boundaries to include partners that have not been previously included in planning and decision-making.

Unite for Sight is a marvelous example of social entrepreneurship:

> "Social entrepreneurs combine best practices in entrepreneurship with a sense of social mission. Creative and innovative, social entrepreneurs are dedicated to improving lives and communities through sustainable social ventures. They step in where the market system has failed to provide for the poor, investing in the development and provision of basic amenities such as health care. They develop high-impact social interventions to lift communities out of poverty and, in Unite For Sight's case, to eliminate preventable blindness worldwide. Our partner eye clinics are led

continues

continued

> *by seasoned social entrepreneurs who organize outreach teams that actively seek out patients in remote villages who would otherwise not have access to eye care. They collaborate with community leaders, governmental bodies, and hospitals to bring high-quality eye care to those living in extreme poverty." (Unite for Sight, n.d., "Social entrepreneurship is at the core of Unite For Sight's working philosophy")*

Organizational Benefits of Partnership

A partnership-based organization is not an unrealistic dream. Organizations exist today that effectively and efficiently provide services and are committed to doing so via partnership. Eisler's (n.d.) research demonstrates the benefits that these organizations experience:

- Employees feel valued and empowered to contribute and participate.

- Conflict can be used creatively to explore alternatives and challenge the status quo.

- Creativity is nurtured through safety for risk taking, less fear of making mistakes, and permission to be inquisitive and explorative.

- Communication is free to flow in all directions—all members of the organization are respected and encouraged to communicate ideas and contribute feedback.

- The workplace is family-friendly, creating a synergistic sense of community.

- Synergistic belonging extends to the planet, creating the social and environmental consciousness needed for long-range planning, sustainability, and success. (Eisler, n.d., Organizational Benefits of Partnership Systems)

For health care—especially community care—these benefits are priceless. They contribute to and nurture the entire system.

Partnership Exemplar: Buurtzorg Nederland (Netherlands Neighborhood-Care)

There is a growing movement toward partnership-based community care, and one of the most noteworthy examples is *Buurtzorg Nederland* (Netherlands Neighborhood-care). Founded in 2006 by Jos de Blok, a district home care nurse and manager, *Buurtzorg Nederland* was a response to the rising threat that the business model poses to community nursing.

In the traditional business model of health care, services are fragmented and assigned to individuals with the lowest level of education and salary. According to de Blok (n.d.), this "product-oriented approach" requires complex systems of coordination and multiple layers of middle management, which contributes to unsustainable systems of health care. Commenting on the impact of the domination system and the alienation that nurses experience, de Blok (n.d.) writes:

> *I entered the healthcare sector out of passion and compassion. I very much wanted to add something to the lives of others. District nurses don't have a job, they are their job. Over the past few years, that has seemed to disappear. Providing care had become something entirely different. It was suddenly all about production, protocols and administration. It was heading in the wrong direction. (p. 2)*

Because de Blok's values were grounded on the nursing story and the full potential of nursing's medicine, he recognized that he was being pushed away from his core. Instead of becoming a victim of a domination system, de Blok designed an alternative model of community care based on partnership principles. He started with one team of nurses in 2007. By 2013, almost 6,000 nurses were employed throughout the country in 580 teams, taking care of 60,000 patients a year (de Blok, personal communication, May 5, 2013).

de Blok's nurses are well educated, with nearly 65% having a baccalaureate degree (p. 83). This allows *Buurtzorg Nederland* to provide care for clients who have a wide variety of complex conditions. Unlike Medicare's restrictive admission criteria, *Buurtzorg Nederland* nurses are able to care for:

- Patients who are terminally ill

- Patients who come from the hospital after surgery, have cancer, and the like

- Patients who have chronic diseases

- Patients who have dementia

- Patients in vulnerable situations with comorbidity (de Blok, 2011, p. 84)

Many more people receive the services they need to remain in their own homes. In fact, the *Buurtzorg Nederland* model has been so successful that it is being implemented for child care, psychiatric home care, and domestic care (de Blok, personal communication, May 5, 2013).

All this is very different from the domination philosophy, which requires Medicare clients to meet rigid homebound requirements. Indeed, *Buurtzorg Nederland* offers a viable model for a partnership approach in every nation's health care system, with great benefits not only to patients and their families but to the finances of government health care systems as well. According to de Blok (2011):

> *The nurses of Buurtzorg see it as their professional duty to enable patients to lead a normal, independent life as long as possible. So they use all the available resources in the environment of the patient, including family, neighbors, or even volunteers to make patients less reliant on the nurses' care. (p. 84)*

In the partnership-based *Buurtzorg Nederland* model, nurses who promote client independence (rather than dependence) provide effective high-quality care. True to partnership systems, the *Buurtzorg Nederland* structure does not promote hierarchies of domination. de Blok (2011) describes the design:

Teams with a maximum of 12 nurses take care of a neighborhood of 15,000 residents, working closely with the GPs and other primary health care workers such as social workers, physiotherapists, ergotherapists, psychiatric nurses, and informal caregivers. An average team supports between 40 and 60 patients at a time. The nurses take care of the assessment, planning, and coordination of the patient care and discuss the continuity with one another. Every patient has a personal guide. In weekly meetings the nurses discuss the patients, the cooperation with others, and the organization of their work. There is no leader within the teams; they work on the basis of consent. Everyone has to take responsibility .... The organization's philosophy is that you don't need to control professionals; all relationships are based on trust and respect. (pp. 84-85)

Buurtzorg Nederland is supported by a very effective web-based infrastructure, called Buurtzorgweb, that also allows nurses to work on certain tasks from home. In describing the impact of their web system, de Blok wrote the following:

The nurses can log in when they want—some do the administration in the evening at home. They can find all the information they need on the Buurtzorgweb and communicate with colleagues from other teams. On different patient groups there are expert groups— nurses who have a certain specialization and develop standards for Buurtzorg as a whole. The web works as a real community. (p. 85)

The web allows the nurses to connect and obtain the information they need when they need it. It also allows them more flexibility in their hours and more time in their own homes. In addition to providing quality care, the partnership-based structure of *Buurtzorg Nederland* is cost effective and delivers maximum quality. de Blok (2011) describes an organization that runs so efficiently it has no managers, and 20 employees in the office can support all the nurses in the field. This low overhead allows *Buurtzorg Nederland* to be very cost-effective. For example, in 2012, the revenues for *Buurtzorg Nederland*, a nonprofit business, were €180 million ($234 million) with a profit of €13 million ($16 million) (de Blok, personal communication, May 5, 2013).

Similarly, *Buurtzorg Nederland* demonstrates that quality care can thrive in a partnership-based model:

- *Buurtzorg Nederland* received the 2011 and 2012 Employer of the Year award in the Netherlands. This award reflects all employers, not just health care.

- On a scale of 10, *Buurtzorg Nederland* consistently received a score of 9.1 for customer satisfaction.

- In 2013, every nurse had the necessary tools to support his or her work on a daily basis, including personal iPads and the Omaha System to help document patient care. (de Blok, personal communication, May 5, 2013)

This data demonstrates that increased client satisfaction and increased nurse engagement work hand in hand to drive *Buurtzorg Nederland*'s exemplary success.

Similar to other partnership-based organizations, leaders in *Buurtzorg Nederland* are facilitators or coaches:

When a new team is starting, the coach helps this team to recruit new colleagues, learn to use the Buurtzorgweb, divide the different roles in the team, and build their network with other caregivers, both formal and informal. In this way every team learns how to deal with problems it faces and develop an excellent, mature team. The role of the coach is also to support the teams so that they can find their own solutions. Each team is different and may have different solutions. (de Blok, 2011, p. 85)

Buurtzorg Nederland's emphasis on autonomy, creativity, and self-organization yields a high level of satisfaction for the nurses. In fact, the *Buurtzorg Nederland* model resonates so deeply with the core of nursing that whole teams of nurses from other home care agencies transfer to *Buurtzorg Nederland*. de Blok (n.d.) summarizes, "If you do something precisely the way it is meant to be done, it can, I believe, hardly fail. District nurses and healthcare workers apply to us spontaneously. We have never had to do any active marketing" (p. 3).

Conclusion

This inspiring story of Jos de Blok and the *Burrtzorg Nederland* nurses demonstrates what can happen when nurses challenge domination-based systems. When nurses implement flatter, less rigid hierarchical structures, promote leadership based on facilitation and coaching, share power or use power with the people they serve, participate in effective teamwork, and dare to be creative social entrepreneurs, anything is possible.

References

Ashoka. (n.d.). What is a social entrepreneur? Retrieved from https://www.ashoka.org/social_entrepreneur

Centers for Medicare & Medicaid Services. (n.d.). Medicare and home health care. Retrieved from http://www.medicare.gov/Pubs/pdf/10969.pdf

Centers for Medicare & Medicaid Services. (2013). Accountable care organizations (ACO). Retrieved from http://www.cms.gov/Medicare/Medicare-Fee-for-Service-Payment/ACO/index.html?redirect=/aco/

Chen, C. Y., Harrington, A., Lustgarten, A., Mero, J., & Tkaczyk, C. (2004). 50 best companies for minorities. Retrieved from http://money.cnn.com/magazines/fortune/fortune_archive/2004/06/28/374393/

de Blok, J. (n.d.). Buurtzorg Nederland. Retrieved from omahasystemmn.org/documents/2010-10-04ArtikelBuurtzorgInHetEngels.pdf

de Blok, J. (2011, Summer). Buurtzorg Nederland: A new perspective on elder care in the Netherlands. *The Journal*, 82-86. Retrieved from http://omahasystem.org/AARPTheJournal_Summer2011_deBlok.pdf

Eisler, R. (n.d.). Organizational benefits of partnership systems. Retrieved from http://www.partnershipway.org/core-pathways/abcs-of-dominator-and-partnership-relations/two-social-possibilities-the-domination-system-and-the-partnership-system

Eisler, R. (1987). *The chalice and the blade: Our history, our future.* San Francisco: CA: Harper & Row.

Eisler, R. (2002). *The power of partnership: Seven relationships that will change your life.* Novato, CA: New World Library.

Eisler, R., & Montuori, A. (2001). The partnership organization: A systems approach. *OD Practitioner, 33*(2), 11-17.

Health Resources and Services Administration (HRSA). (2010). *Registered nurse population: Findings from the 2008 national sample survey of registered nurses.* Washington, DC: Department of Health and Human Services.

Human Resource in a Nutshell. (2011). OD practitioner. Retrieved from http://www. hrnutshell.com/topics/topics-covered-group1-key-to-survival/change-mgt/item/232-od-practitioner

Institute for Healthcare Improvement (IHI). (2013). IHI triple aim initiative. Retrieved from http://www.ihi.org/offerings/Initiatives/TripleAim/Pages/default.aspx

Institute of Medicine (IOM). (2010). *The future of nursing: Leading change, advancing health.* (Report brief). Washington, DC: National Academies.

MacWilliams, R. B., Schmidt, B., & Bleich, M. R. (2013). Men in nursing: Understanding the challenges men face working in a predominantly female profession. *AJN, 113*(1), 38-44.

Mayes, R. (2007). The origins, development, and passage of Medicare's revolutionary prospective payment system. *Journal of the History of and Allied Sciences, 62*(1), 21-55. doi: 10.1093/jhmas/jrj038

Potter, T. M. (2013). *The BASE of nursing.* Unpublished manuscript, School of Nursing, University of Minnesota, United States of America.

Unite for Sight. (n. d.). Social entrepreneurship is at the core of Unite For Sight's working philosophy. Retrieved from http://www.uniteforsight.org/what-we-do/social-entrepreneurship

United States Census Bureau. (2012). U.S. census bureau projections show a slower growing, older, more diverse nation a half century from now. Retrieved from https://www.census.gov/newsroom/releases/archives/population/cb12-243.html

United States Census Bureau. (2013). Male nurses becoming more common place census bureau reports. Retrieved from https://www.census.gov/newsroom/releases/archives/employment_occupations/cb13-32.html

World Health Organization (WHO). (2008). *Taking stock: Task shifting to tackle health worker shortages.* Geneva, Switzerland: Health Systems and Services.

Chapter 12
Patterns of Partnership and Domination in the Nursing-Nature Relationship

"Nature alone cures. Surgery removes the bullet out of the limb, which is an obstruction to cure, but nature heals the wound. So it is with medicine; the function of an organ becomes obstructed; medicine, so far as we know, assists nature to remove the obstruction, but does nothing more. And what nursing has to do in either case is to put the patient in the best condition for nature to act upon him."

–Florence Nightingale, 1860 (1969, p. 133)

Eisler partnered with Daniel S. Levine, a professor in the field of psychology and neuroscience, to explore the science behind a possible genetic link between genes, cultural environments, and caring or uncaring behaviors. In their article

"Nurture, Nature, and Caring: We Are Not Prisoners of our Genes" (2002), the authors describe the interplay of biology (genetics) and social environments (experiences), and offer this challenge:

> *The yearning by both men and women for caring connections, for peace rather than war, for equality rather than inequality, for freedom rather than oppression, can be seen as part of the human genetic equipment. The degree to which this yearning can be realized is not a matter of changing our genes, but of building social structures and systems of belief that support rather than inhibit the human capacity for caring. (Eisler & Levine, 2002, p. 46)*

We are not simply puppets controlled by evolutionary genetic imperatives, as some popular sociobiologists and evolutionary psychologists claim. Nor do we have to blindly continue the once hallowed "conquest of nature"—another tradition of domination that threatens to destroy our natural life-support systems.

NPR journalist Thom Hartmann (2004) describes the broken belief system that has led to our current estranged relationship with nature. In *Last Hours of Ancient Sunlight: The Fate of the World and What We Can Do Before It's Too Late,* Hartmann warns of dire implications of the current cultural story, including mass extinction and ecosystem degradation. Like Eisler in *The Chalice and the Blade* (1987), Hartmann (2004) argues that the current destructive story is relatively new: "This shrinking into separateness, this breaking of the intimate bond with the world around us, this separating ourselves into isolated 'boxes,' was largely unknown for the first 100,000 years or more of human history" (p. 133). He too proposes this new cultural story is a usurper, an interloper on a more ancient and healthier cultural story.

Hartmann (2004) notes that ancient indigenous communities around the globe frequently based their beliefs and values on a partnership story or cultural narrative. This is not to say that all indigenous cultures were, or are, partnership cultures—there were, and still are, indigenous cultures that orient closely to the domination model. However, his study of literature from anthropology led

Hartmann (2004) to conclude that there was an ancient partnership story that allowed many communities to have the following:

> [M]ore leisurely lives, less poverty, almost no crime, a more diverse and healthy diet, less degenerative disease, better psychological health, and a culture that holds as its primary values cooperation (rather than competition), mutual respect (rather than domination), long-term renewable care for resources (rather than exploitation for a quick buck), and equality (between people, between the sexes, and between humans and nature) rather than power. (p. 175)

As discussed in Chapter 3, there is even today a very different story about nature among more partnership-oriented cultures such as the Minangkabau (Sanday, 2002). The story bears repeating here:

> The Minangkabau weave order out of their version of wild nature by appealing to maternal archetypes. Unlike Darwin in the 19th century, the Minangkabau subordinate male dominion and competition, which we consider basic to human social ordering and evolution, to the work of maternal nurture, which they hold to be necessary for the common good and the healthy society ... Social well-being is found in natural growth and fertility according to the dictum that the unfurling, blooming, and growth in nature is our teacher. (2002, pp. 22-24)

Both Eisler (1987, 2002) and Hartmann (2004) propose that many of our current problems are related to the domination story that has shaped our beliefs, our values, and our perception of reality. This cultural story is unconsciously transmitted from generation to generation and will only change as we question and refute it.

The nursing profession has been noticeably absent from the discussion of cultural stories about nature, yet the prevalent cultural story directly impacts nursing and health care in dramatic ways. It impacts the quality of our relationship with nature and, therefore, according to Nightingale (1969) and other earlier nurses, our full potential for health and healing. Therefore, nurses need to examine domination-based cultural assumptions about nature.

Identifying Domination Challenges in the Nursing-Nature Relationship

As explained earlier, nursing's roots are embedded in a deep commitment and respect for nature as a healer. Many nurses and other healers worked in partnership with nature. Today, most nurses barely give a passing nod to the role that nature plays in healing.

SELECTED RESEARCH RELATED TO NATURE'S ROLE IN HEALING

In 1984, Robert Ulrich became one of the first researchers to study the healing impact of nature. He studied the outcomes of 46 cholecystectomy patients with similar demographics. Half had rooms with windows looking out on a natural scene. The other half of the patients had rooms with windows facing a brick wall. The patients who were able to look out at a natural scene required less pain medication, registered fewer complaints in the nurses' notes, and were discharged sooner than the patients without a natural view. The same results today would have significant implications for Hospital Consumer Assessment of Healthcare Providers and Systems (HCAPS) scores.

More recently, Astell-Burt, Feng, and Kolt (2013) did a cross-data analysis of over 250,000 Australians over age 45 with valid sleep data. Sleep plays a significant role in chronic illness, wound healing, psychological health, and prevention of obesity and, therefore, is of concern.

Results of the study demonstrated that the prevalence of sleep for 8 or more hours correlated with living in neighborhoods with more green space. Sleeping less than 8 hours correlated with neighborhoods with less green space. Green space appears to impact health regardless of other factors including socio-economic status and physical activity.

The authors conclude, "Green space planning policies may have wider public health benefits than previously recognized." (p. 1)

It must be emphasized that partnership with nature does *not* mean abandoning the knowledge and tools that help us heal from illnesses or accidents. Indeed, many diagnostic and treatment advances for conditions that in the past would have maimed or killed must be valued and used—and in a more partnership-oriented world will be made available to many people who are denied them today.

However, many current health problems are directly related to a domination perspective of nature, as illustrated by the following examples:

- Indiscriminant use of antibiotics and other antimicrobials (in both humans and animals) resulting in multidrug-resistant organisms

- Health problems related to the disposal of vast amounts of medical waste

- Overuse of antibacterial soaps

- Health issues related to climate change

Each of these problems is complex and involves many factors, but the domination paradigm is a major commonality.

Indiscriminant Use of Antibiotics

Antibiotics have been important medical tools, preventing many deaths worldwide. But the indiscriminate, excessive use of antibiotics and other antimicrobials has created new health problems and led to unnecessary deaths. The notion has backfired that by using more "medical weapons" we can "conquer" nature. The organisms that the "weapons" were designed to eradicate have, in a sense, outsmarted us.

In his testimony before the U.S. Congress, Stuart Levy (2010), professor at Tufts University School of Medicine and president of the Alliance for the Prudent Use of Antibiotics (APUA), blamed the current epidemic of multidrug-resistant organisms on the misuse of antimicrobials in both human medicine and animal agriculture. He pointed to the following health implications of antibiotic resistance:

- Increased difficulty finding effective treatments

- Increased health care costs related to increased hospital length-of-stays and the need for more expensive drugs to successfully treat infections

- The rise of hospital acquired infections (HAIs)

- Death of patients when all antibiotic options have been exhausted (Levy & Marshall, 2004)

Here is an instance where the notion that humans can "conquer" nature, combined with an economic system that is still largely guided by lack of care for people and nature (Chapter 13), has led to problems that could have been avoided in a more partnership-oriented system.

Medical Waste Disposal

It is quite ironic that the industry whose mission it is to prevent and treat illness is also one of the largest contributors to environmentally caused diseases. According to Heilprin (2011), estimates indicate wealthy nations generate up to 13 pounds and poorer nations up to 6.6 pounds per person per year of hazardous medical waste. This waste contains pathogens, blood, low levels of radioactivity, discarded needles, syringes, scalpels, and expired drugs and vaccines. Heilprin also notes that in many poorer nations, discarded chemicals and pharmaceutical wastes go straight to city dumps, down hospital toilets into water systems, or are burned in cement kilns that add to dioxide emissions.

Hazardous wastes that get into the environment pose numerous risks. The World Health Organization (WHO, 2011) lists the following health-related risks:

- Harmful microorganisms that can affect patients, health care workers, and the general public

- Radiation burns

- Sharps-inflicted injuries

- Poisoning and pollution through the release of pharmaceutical products (in particular, antibiotics and cytotoxic drugs)

- Poisoning and pollution through waste water

- Poisoning and pollution by toxins such as mercury or dioxins that are released during incineration of waste products ("Health impact" section)

Wealthier nations generally incinerate most of their medical waste to keep it out of landfills and groundwater, but incineration carries health risks. For example, the health care industry produces over 4 billion pounds of waste each year, most of it in the form of plastics. Dioxins are released when PVC plastics are incinerated, and "research has linked dioxins with cancer, reproductive and developmental problems, chloracne, and endocrine and immune disorders" (Melamed & Wilburn, 2001). Mercury is also released during incineration, and it is shown to impact the neurological development of fetuses and children (Environmental Protection Agency [EPA], 2012).

Chapter 13 explores this problem and how it is directly related to both an ethos of domination and an economic system focused on short-term monetary profits (rather than long-term planning that ensures that people and habitat are cared for and protected).

Antibacterial Soaps Containing Triclosan

There is growing recognition of the issue of groundwater contamination by pharmaceuticals and personal care products. For instance, the United States Geological Survey (USGS) found low levels of drugs such as antibiotics, hormones, contraceptives, and steroids in 80% of the rivers and streams they tested between 1999 and 2000 (USGS, 2002).

One of the chemicals currently being scrutinized by the U.S. Food and Drug Administration (FDA) is *triclosan*. Even though the Environmental Protection Agency (EPA) has registered the chemical as a pesticide (EPA, 2010), triclosan is added to many consumer products to decrease or prevent bacterial contamination. According to the Food and Drug Administration (FDA, 2012) triclosan is found in household products such as clothing, toys, furniture, and items used for cooking. It also may be added to personal hygiene products, including antibacterial soaps, body washes, toothpastes, and cosmetics. Studies show that triclosan alters hormone regulation in animals and contributes to antibiotic resistance (FDA, 2012). Triclosan has also been found to significantly impact cardiac muscle contractility in animals (Cherednichenko et al., 2012).

Interestingly, aside from triclosan's ability to decrease the risk of gingivitis when used in toothpastes, the FDA (2012) concludes, "At this time, the agency does not have evidence that triclosan in antibacterial soaps and body washes provides any benefit over washing with regular soap and water" ("Does triclosan provide a benefit in consumer products?" section).

If triclosan poses significant known risks in animals and potentially severe risks in humans, why is triclosan still used in products we rub on our skin and in toys that children put in their mouths? The answer lies in the domination system of beliefs and values. As will be discussed in Chapter 13, this system has led to ways of measuring economic productivity that do not take into account the damage to people and nature caused by some of this "productivity."

Climate Change and Its Impact on Health

The popular media frequently make statements suggesting that scientists don't agree about the cause of global climate change (McKelway, 2013). This ignores what the overwhelming majority of scientists tell us, as shown in this report from a U.S. government agency: "Ninety-seven percent of climate scientists agree that climate-warming trends over the past century are very likely due to human activities, and most of the leading scientific organizations worldwide have issued public statements endorsing this position" (National Aeronautics and Space Administration [NASA], n.d.).

Signs of climate change are apparent in rising sea levels, droughts and floods, poor air quality, intense tropical storms, hurricanes and tornados, and profound heat waves. The health implications related to climate change are clear—and dire. The WHO (2012) describes the following severe health impacts:

- Climate change affects the social and environmental determinants of health—clean air, safe drinking water, sufficient food, and secure shelter.

- Since the 1970s, over 140,000 additional deaths each year can be attributed to global warming.

- The direct damage costs to health (excluding costs in health-determining sectors such as agriculture, water, and sanitation) by 2030 are estimated as between 2–4 billion U.S. dollars per year.

- Many of the major killers, such as diarrheal diseases, malnutrition, malaria, and dengue are highly climate sensitive and are expected to worsen as the climate changes. ("Key facts" section)

The EPA (2013) warns that climate change is already increasing pollution and pollen, resulting in a rise of severe respiratory illnesses. We are also more likely to see increases in food-borne, water-borne, and animal-borne diseases in the years ahead. In addition, the Centers for Disease Control and Prevention (CDC, 2013) has prepared an Extreme Heat Communication Toolkit for public health workers in anticipation of severe heat outbreaks that pose particular hazards for vulnerable people such as the elderly, small children, and homeless people.

All this information is readily available. Why has it had so little impact on public attitudes and government policies? The answer lies in one of the most common aspects of the domination mindset: *denial*. As Eisler (2002) writes, people raised in families with the domination perspective—families where they learn that the adults on whom they depend for their survival may not be contradicted—tend to have a hard time contradicting what their "superiors" tell them, even when they are adults. They therefore tend to:

- Find it difficult to question, much less challenge, powerful economic interests on whom they feel dependent

- Have difficulty looking at the long-range future

- Place emphasis on the short-term bottom line because they're stuck in a defensive mode of protecting themselves and what they have

- Have trouble dealing with change (p. 161)

In health care, this denial can be seen in our refusal to believe that we will ever run out of antibiotic options to treat resistant strains of microorganisms.

Denial is evident when health care providers appear oblivious to the impact of medical waste on the environment. Health care consumers are also in a state of denial when they refuse to acknowledge the risks associated with overuse of antibacterial products. Policymakers and the constituents who support them are also in denial when they refuse to acknowledge global climate change.

Part of the problem is that products and processes that can cause tremendous harm to the environment are billed as normal and nothing to be concerned about by powerful economic players. Those players benefit from this kind psychic numbing (or more accurately, *psychic norming*). The counter-messaging about climate change is one of the most glaring examples of this phenomenon, reinforcing the tendency of many people to ignore what would otherwise be obvious. In other words, these messages tend to make the general public numb to climate change science, allowing policymakers to refuse to significantly reduce fossil fuel use—despite overwhelming evidence that we are on a rapid path to extinction due to climate change.

If humans are to survive on this planet, the domination system must be challenged. The old stories must be replaced with a new paradigm that supports a more sustainable, caring way of living and making a living. Nurses can play an important role in this paradigm shift.

An Alternative Partnership Approach in the Nursing-Nature Relationship

For nurses to reclaim a life-sustaining relationship with nature, we need to first deconstruct and challenge myths embedded in the domination story. If we don't challenge these myths, it is difficult to create and sustain a new story.

Three domination myths particularly inhibit a healthy nurse-nature relationship:

1. Humans and nature are separate.

2. Humans are ranked far above nature in the hierarchy of importance.

3. It is moral, just, and therefore good to use our natural resources based solely on the current needs of humanity. The needs of future generations are of no concern when there are so many pressing needs today.

These myths are major obstacles to change. This is why recovering our lost relationship with nature does not just entail replacing our incandescent light bulbs with compact florescent bulbs. It requires that we replace the cultural stories and assumptions that broke our relationship in the first place with a partnership story that works.

The medicine of nursing and the BASE of Nursing (Potter, 2013) position nurses to actualize partnership-based values in health care. The partnership-based belief system is built on the following values and nursing actions related to nature:

- Humans and nature are indivisible. We are one interconnected whole.

- Humans and nature are in a partnership-based relationship.

- We must ask, "How will my actions as a nurse impact future generations?"

Humans and Nature Are Indivisible

What we do to one part of the natural system directly impacts the health of the entire system. Therefore, it is *essential* for nurses to consider every action's positive *and* negative implications.

Philosopher and ecologist David Abram (1996) poetically describes the deeper ways of perceiving that were normative for many of our ancestors. In *The Spell of the Sensuous*, Abram explains that the survival of humanity depended on our ancestors' acute and accurate perception of the environment; hence, the margins of the human body were more fluid and open.

The breathing, sensing body draws its sustenance and its very substance from the soils, plants, and elements that surround it; it continually contributes itself, in turn, to the air, to the composting earth, to the nourishment of insects and oak trees and squirrels, ceaselessly spreading out of itself as well as breathing the world into itself, so that it is very difficult to discern, at any moment, precisely where this living body begins and where it ends. (pp. 46-47)

Potter and Peden-McAlpine (2002) similarly explain the phenomenon of *early recognition*, a skill frequently used by expert nurses in the field. In addition, Potter's (2010) research demonstrated that acute observation, early recognition, and other ways of knowing were common themes in the autobiographies of historic partnership nurses. Perception and acute observation are therefore part of *being present* in the BASE of Nursing (Potter, 2013).

Sample actions to shift and deepen your partnership with nature when you nurse:

- Begin every patient/client relationship with the understanding that you are connecting to a whole. You will be in a relationship with not only the patient's bodymindspirit, but also the bodymindspirit of their families and the patient's entire social support network.

- Listen for narratives that reveal the patient's connections or lack of connections to the whole. Are the strands of the web of life that link them to their families solid and strong, or are they weak and broken? Do they have strands connecting them to friends? How many? What is the nature of these strands: weak, strong, conditionally present? Is the patient connected to the community? Are these community strands weak or strong?

- What does the patient do to maintain a connection to the rest of nature? How often is she or he in nature? What aspects of nature hold specific "medicine" for them? Does the ocean, a walk in the forest, a mountain view, renew the patient? Does the patient make lifestyle choices that harm or weaken his or her relationship with nature? What can the patient do to strengthen these strands?

- As a nurse, you can teach patients how to assess the strength of their own strands. The nurse can teach patients how to strengthen weak strands. The nurse can also make referrals or facilitate connections to services that can help patients strengthen their web of life.

Humans and Nature Are in a Partnership-Based Relationship

Instead of having dominion over nature, we can seek to be in a hierarchy of actualization with nature, where any power we have is used to empower and support the entire biosphere.

Sample actions to shift and deepen your partnership with nature:

- Carefully observe signs and symptoms. Instead of viewing them as something to be controlled and suppressed (domination logic), view them as communication from the patients' bodymindspirit. What is the bodymindspirit trying to tell you? What message do the signs or symptoms convey? Are there unmet needs underlying the current signs and symptoms? Are there imbalances that need to be rebalanced by supportive interventions? What can you do to put the patient in the best place for nature to heal itself?

- Nurses can watch for subtle pattern shifts that may occur before lab results change significantly or before technology warns us. These shifts are frequently the earliest indications that the patient is entering a state of imbalance and should be brought to the attention of the interprofessional team.

The unique medicine of nursing resides in nurses' presence and receptivity to narrative data. Spending more time in direct contact with the client makes subtle shifts or patient status changes more obvious to the nurse. You can recognize imbalances sooner so more effective, less costly interventions can be implemented (Potter & Peden-McAlpine, 2002).

How Will My Actions as a Nurse Impact Future Generations?

Consideration of future generations is not a new idea; you can find it around the globe in many indigenous cultures. For example, consider the Great Binding Law of the Iroquois Confederacy, a Native American nation in the northeast United States. Scholars believe their oral law may have influenced the drafting of the Constitution of the United States (Halsall, 1997). The Great Binding Law states the following:

> *In all of your deliberations in the Confederate Council, in your efforts at law making, in all your official acts, self-interest shall be cast into oblivion. Cast not over your shoulder behind you the warnings of the nephews and nieces should they chide you for any error or wrong you may do, but return to the way of the Great Law, which is just and right. Look and listen for the welfare of the whole people and have always in view not only the present but also the coming generations, even those whose faces are yet beneath the surface of the ground—the unborn of the future Nation. (Halsall, 1997, Article 28)*

Sample actions to promote a sustainable relationship with nature:

- In every action, partnership nurses are mindful of the environmental implications. How much waste are you generating? How much energy is required to make this intervention possible? Will the intervention impact future generations? If the intervention potentially harms future generations, is there an equally effective alternative that is not harmful?

- To protect future generations, become involved on a system-wide level. Offer to be on the product procurement committee or the waste management committee for the health care organization where you work.

- Pursue excellence in the emerging field of integrative nursing, which has the following nature-based principles:

  - Human beings are whole systems inseparable from their environment.

- Human beings have the innate capacity for health and well-being across all the dimensions (bodymindspirit).

- Nature has healing and restorative properties that contribute to health and well-being. (Kreitzer & Koithan, 2014)

These three core values and principles can help nurses shift the current health care system's paradigm away from domination toward partnership.

Partnership-Based Exemplar: Health Care Without Harm

The nonprofit organization Health Care Without Harm (HCWH) is an excellent exemplar of an organization that brings health care stakeholders together for the purpose of reducing our harm to the environment. Stakeholders include an international coalition of hospitals and health care systems, health care providers and staff, environmental health organizations, community groups, labor unions, religious groups, and communities impacted by health care practices related to the environment. The mission of Health Care Without Harm is to "Transform the health care sector worldwide, without compromising patient safety or care, so that it is ecologically sustainable and no longer a source of harm to public health and the environment" (Health Care Without Harm, n.d.).

HCWH's goal is to shift policies and procedures toward health for both humans and the environment. The official website states:

The huge scale of the health care sector worldwide means that unhealthy practices—such as poor waste management, use of toxic chemicals, unhealthy food choices and reliance on polluting technologies—have a major negative impact on the health of humans and the environment. The good news is that the health care sector can play a leading role in solving these problems. Due to its massive buying power, and its mission-driven interest in preventing disease, the health care sector can help shift the entire economy toward sustainable, safer products and practices. (Health Care Without Harm, n.d.)

Health Care Without Harm has eight core goals:

- Create markets and policies for safer products and materials in health care.

- Eliminate incineration of medical wastes.

- Design health care facilities to have minimal impact on the environment and to truly be healing environments.

- Encourage purchasing of sustainable and healthy foods that cause no harm to the health of patients and employees.

- Create a safe and healthy workplace.

- Be totally transparent about the chemical contents of all materials so employees and patients can make informed decisions about their use.

- Promote human rights and environmental justice for all people so that problems are not relocated from one community to another.

- Battle climate change with improved energy practices and a reduced overall health care carbon footprint. (Health Care Without Harm, n.d.)

Health care organizations are invited to use HCWH's information, expertise, and frameworks for action in their own communities. There is no membership fee for organizations to join HCWH.

In fewer than 10 years, Health Care Without Harm's global membership has successfully launched several initiatives that improve the health of the human-nature connection:

- Eliminating mercury in medical products and equipment

- Closing thousands of medical waste incinerators around the world

- Starting a green building program for health care organizations

- Developing a healthy food program

- Creating programs to decrease the carbon footprint of the health care system (Health Care Without Harm, n.d.)

Another HCWH initiative is *Practice Green Health* (2013), a program co-created with the American Nurses Association. This program allows hospitals and other health care organizations to compete for awards and recognition. The awards demonstrate the organizations' commitment to patient safety and healthy care environments, and they offer a way to attract patients and employees who value a partnership with nature.

Conclusion

Nurses and other health professionals are beginning to boldly claim a new relationship with nature. Based on a partnership system of beliefs, health professionals around the globe are beginning to remember and honor the ancient understanding that nature can be the healer and that their role (our role) is to be supportive partners.

The next chapter turns to an indispensable component for building partnership-based health care and a partnership society: a caring economics that gives visibility and real value to the work of caring for both people and nature.

FACILITATING NATURE AS HEALER

Nurses can do several things to partner with nature's ability to heal:

- *Examine your language, making sure when you refer to nature you use partnership language rather than domination language. For example: "working with disease" rather than "fighting disease" and "supporting the bacteria that help our body function" rather than always being antibacteria.*

- *Facilitate opportunities for patients to be exposed to fresh air, natural plants, and sunshine.*

- *When doing a health assessment, routinely ask about the amount of time a client spends in nature. This can open further dialogue and teaching about the important role nature plays in healing.*

continues

continued

- *Teach parents the importance of having children regularly play out-doors. Richard Louv's (2008)* Last Child in the Woods: Saving Our Children from Nature-Deficit Disorder *is a wonderful resource for patient education.*

- *Role-model a healthy relationship with nature by walking, biking, and spending time outdoors as part of your own self-care routine.*

- *Teach patients to take every single antibiotic dose that they have been prescribed (to prevent development of resistance).*

- *Teach patients to read food labels and to select products where antibiotics have not been used in production of the food.*

- *Teach patients and families that good hand washing with normal soap is sufficient for preventing most infections. Antibacterial soap is not necessary in everyday use unless there are issues related to immune compromise.*

- *Volunteer to be on hospital supply committees to make sure that purchased products are Energy Star-rated, come with the least amount of packaging, are made of recycled paper or plastics where possible, and have as low an environmental impact as possible. Regularly ask if a product will harm future generations.*

- *Facilitate your hospital or clinic enrolling to be members of Health Care Without Harm. Work on initiatives so that your organization can apply for one of the Practice Green awards and be recognized for its commitment to the environment.*

- *Review policies and procedures to be certain they support environmental health and sustainability.*

- *Request that your hospital/clinic install motion detector lights in all the patient rooms, bathrooms, and supply closets.*

- *Before purchasing or using a product, stop and ask if it is really necessary.*

- *Teach patients about the wonder of the human body: how the systems work together, the amazing complexity, and the unimaginable beauty of processes (such as wound healing) often taken for granted.*

- *Work at a state and national level for health policies that do not harm nature.*

- *Encourage everyone to decrease the carbon footprint in our homes and places we work.*

- *Write and speak out so communities know that nurses partner with nature to create environments for healing.*

References

Abram, D. (1996). *The spell of the sensuous.* New York, NY: Vintage Books.

Astell-Burt, T., Feng, X., & Kolt, G. S. (2013). Does access to neighbourhood green space promote a healthy duration of sleep? Novel findings from a cross-sectional study of 259 319 Australians. *British Medical Journal [BMJ] Open 3,* 1-6. doi: 10.1136/bmjopen-2013-003094

Centers for Disease Control and Prevention (CDC). (2013). Public health response to a changing climate. Retrieved from http://www.cdc.gov/features/changingclimate/

Cherednichenko, G., Zhang, R., Bannister, R. A., Timofeyev, V., Li, N., Fritsch, E. B.,... Pessah, I. N. (2012). Triclosan impairs excitation-contraction coupling and Ca2+ dynamics in striated muscle. *Proceedings of the National Academy of Sciences, 109*(35). Online publication. doi:10.1073/pnas.1211314109

Eisler, R. (1987). *The chalice and the blade: Our history and our future.* San Francisco, CA: HarperCollins.

Eisler, R. (2002). *The power of partnership: Seven relationships that will change your life.* Novato, CA: New World Library.

Eisler, R., & Levine, D. S. (2002). Nurture, nature, and caring: We are not prisoners of our genes. *Brain and Mind, 3,* 9-52.

Environmental Protection Agency (EPA). (2010). Triclosan facts. Retrieved from http://www.epa.gov/oppsrrd1/REDs/factsheets/triclosan_fs.htm

Environmental Protection Agency (EPA). (2012). Mercury: Health effects. Retrieved from http://www.epa.gov/hg/effects.htm

Environmental Protection Agency (EPA). (2013). Human health impacts and adaptation: Climate change. Retrieved from http://www.epa.gov/climatechange/impacts-adaptation/health.html

Food and Drug Administration (FDA). (2012). Triclosan: What consumers should know. Retrieved from http://www.fda.gov/forconsumers/consumerupdates/ucm205999.htm

Halsall, P. (1997). Modern history sourcebook: The constitution of the Iroquois Confederacy. Retrieved from http://www.fordham.edu/halsall/mod/iroquois.asp

Hartmann, T. (2004). *The last hours of ancient sunlight: The fate of the world and what we can do before it is too late* (Rev. ed.). New York, NY: Three Rivers Press.

Health Care Without Harm. (n.d.). Mission and vision. Retrieved from http://www.noharm.org/all_regions/about/mission.php

Heilprin, J. (2011). Medical waste carries health risks, needs more regulation: U. N. investigator. *Huffington Post.* Retrieved from http://www.huffingtonpost.com/2011/09/14/medical-waste-health-risks_n_962541.html?view=print&comm_ref=false

Kreitzer, M. J., & Koithan, M. (Eds.). (2014). *Integrative nursing.* New York, NY: Oxford Press.

Levy, S. (2010). Testimony before the subcommittee on health of the U.S. House committee on energy and commerce. (July 14, 2010). Retrieved from http://www.tufts.edu/med/apua/policy/7.14.10.pdf

Levy, S., & Marshall, B. (2004). Antibacterial resistance worldwide: Causes, challenges and responses. *Nature Medicine Supplement, 10*(12 Suppl), S122-S129.

Louv, R. (2008). *Last child in the woods: Saving our children from nature-deficit disorder.* New York, NY: Workman Publishing.

McKelway, D. (2013). Climate change skeptics seize on reports showing temperatures leveling. Retrieved from http://www.foxnews.com/politics/2013/04/09/climate-change-skeptics-seize-on-reports-showing-temperatures-leveling/

Melamed, A., & Wilburn, S. (2001). When health care harms: The dangers of incinerating medical waste. *American Journal of Nursing, 101*(4). Retrieved from http://nursingworld.org/MainMenuCategories/WorkplaceSafety/Healthy-Work-Environment/Environmental-Health/Issues/Facility/MedicalWaste/AJNArticle.html?css=print

National Aeronautics and Space Administration (NASA). (n.d.). Global climate change: Vital signs of the planet. Retrieved from http://climate.nasa.gov/scientific-consensus

Nightingale, F. (1969). *Notes on nursing: What it is and what it is not.* New York: Dover.

Potter, T. M. (2010). Reconstructing a new story of nursing: Critical analysis of nursing textbooks using Riane Eisler's partnership paradigm. *Dissertation Abstracts International, 72*(05), 3447086.

Potter, T. M. (2013). *The BASE of nursing.* Unpublished manuscript, School of Nursing, University of Minnesota, United States of America.

Potter, T., & Peden-McAlpine, C. (2002). How expert home care nurses recognize early client status changes. *Home Healthcare Nurse, 20*(1), 43-50.

Practice Green Health. (2013). 2013 Environmental excellence awards. Retrieved from https://practicegreenhealth.org/awards/award-types

Sanday, P. R. (2002). *Women in the center: Life in a modern matriarchy.* Ithaca, NY: Cornell University Press.

Ulrich, R. (1984). View through a window may influence recovery from surgery. *Science 224*(4647), 420-421.

United States Geological Survey (USGS). (2002). Pharmaceuticals, hormones, and other organic wastewater contaminants in U.S. streams. Retrieved from http://toxics.usgs.gov/pubs/FS-027-02/

World Health Organization (WHO). (2011). Waste from health-care activities. Retrieved from http://www.who.int/mediacentre/factsheets/fs253/en/#

World Health Organization (WHO). (2012). Climate change and health. Retrieved from http://www.who.int/mediacentre/factsheets/fs266/en/

Part IV
Next Steps

"Why, when we humans have such a great capacity for caring, consciousness, and creativity, has our world seen so much cruelty, insensitivity, and destructiveness?"

–Riane Eisler, The Real Wealth of Nations, *2007, p. 1*

The final part of this book looks to the future and calls on leaders of every health care profession to step forward and support the full development of partnership-based organizations and economies.

Chapter 13 describes Riane Eisler's caring economics theory and why the shift to a new economic model is essential for improved quality and sustainability of the health care system. Eisler shows how this economic model is far more likely to support the goals and values of health care professionals than models driven solely by financial profit.

The book concludes with **Chapter 14,** which describes specific steps that health care executives, public policy advocates, and professional organizations can take to replace domination structures with partnership-based models of health care.

Our focus in this book has been on the unfolding story of partnership-based health care with a specific look at the nursing profession. But every one of us is needed to shift the health care system away from domination.

Patients and families need to assert their right to be partners. Health care providers need healthy intraprofessional relations and respectful communication that support effective interprofessional practice. Citizens have to hold their local and national governments accountable for implementing economic models that give adequate value and support to the most essential national resource: caring.

Chapter 13
Caring Economics: A Key to Health Care Reform

"We have to change our present economic systems if we, our children, and future generations are to survive and thrive."
—Riane Eisler, The Real Wealth of Nations, *2007, p. 1*

We are not used to thinking of caring and economics together. But what if we did? Would we see so much degradation and despoliation of people and nature, so much poverty and injustice, so much suffering and environmental destruction? Would the work of care continue to be devalued? These questions are especially relevant for the future of health care and the advancement of nursing to its rightful place in both preventing illness and healing. For this reason, even though economics has not traditionally been part of nursing education, we are proposing that it should be.

Learning about economics will help nurses understand health care finance so they can advocate for economic support of effective care models by pointing to how these can also be more cost-effective. We want all nurses to be equipped to understand the shortcomings of conventional economic thinking and become active participants in building a new economic system that recognizes the enormous value of the work of care.

We start this chapter with a premise that, once articulated, may seem self-evident: The real wealth of a nation is not financial. If you think about it, this became painfully obvious with the melting into thin air of all those credit swaps and derivatives during the "Great Recession." Indeed, you can see the ephemeral nature of financial riches every day as stock prices, home prices, and other financial valuations keep seesawing up and down.

The chapter then goes on to one of the main themes in Eisler's 2007 book *The Real Wealth of Nations: Creating a Caring Economics*: that a nation's real wealth consists of the contributions of people and of nature. Therefore, we need what we have not had—economic measurements, policies, and practices that give visibility and adequate value to the most important human work: the work of caring for people, starting in early childhood, and caring for our natural environment.

Nurses, of course, know the enormous value of caring, both for healing people and maintaining good health. But the work of caring is actually integral to all areas of our lives—including economics. Consider this: Without caring and caregiving, none of us would be here. There would be no households, no workforce, no economy, nothing. Especially now, when flexible, creative people who can work in teams and think in long-term ways are essential for economic success, it can be argued that the caring activities still generally categorized as "reproductive work" are actually the most productive activities of all. Similarly, caring for our natural environment is today a prerequisite not only for sustainability, but also for humanity's future survival.

Yet despite all this, most current economic discussions do not mention caring and caregiving. Nor is the value of the work of caring in households included in current economic measurements.

It does not have to be this way. Indeed, the social and economic dislocations inherent in the current shift from the industrial to the postindustrial era offer us an unprecedented opportunity to reexamine and restructure economic theory and practice. Availing ourselves of this opportunity is essential if we are to move to a more equitable, sustainable, and caring future. We know today, from both psychology and neuroscience, that whether or not people are cared for directly impacts human development, health, and life quality. Moreover, moving to an economic system that recognizes the value of care is essential to ensuring that the nursing profession, which is so identified with caring, is given the respect and equality it deserves in new interprofessional health delivery models.

Conventional Economic Thinking

Today, gross domestic product (GDP) is still the primary measurement of economic health. GDP calculates "the monetary value of all the finished goods and services produced within a country's borders in a specific time period." This "includes all of private and public consumption, government outlays, investments and exports less imports that occur within a defined territory" (Investopedia, 2013, "Definition" section).

Policymakers rely heavily on GDP to make the economic decisions that directly affect our lives. Yet GDP disregards poverty, hunger, disease, and environmental degradation. In fact, GDP often goes up at the same time that unemployment, foreclosures, and bankruptcy rates rise. Not only that, GDP gives no indication of the human and environmental damage caused by many activities it includes as "productive." For example, in the United States, where consumer spending accounts for no less than 70% of GDP (Stewart, 2010), much of what is produced and consumed is known to cause disease or even death. This includes the products of multibillion dollar industries ranging from chemical, pesticide, fast food, and packaged food industries to the cigarette, alcohol, and gun industries—all producing "goods" that lead to illness and, with this, to huge medical and funeral costs. In turn, these medical and funeral costs are then also included in GDP as "productivity" (Eisler, 2012).

A significant portion of what is included as productivity in GDP also consists of financial speculations. The U.S. financial sector is now almost 10% of GDP (Schram, 2011), and its value fluctuates wildly—like when trillions of dollars of "wealth" disappeared in the Great Recession of 2008. In this regard, GDP does not reflect the creation of anything that has lasting value, much less a nation's real economic health.

The need for different ways of assessing economic health is further highlighted by the fact that many appliances, electronics, and other products are today deliberately manufactured for planned obsolescence—that is, to break down in a short amount of time so they have to be replaced. This practice is more profitable for manufacturers, but costs consumers a great deal of money they should not have to spend. On top of this, it leads to more clutter in our already bulging landfills.

Current common patterns of production, transportation, and consumption are also often unhealthy for people and nature. For example, emissions from the burning of fossil fuels contribute to rising levels of asthma and other respiratory diseases, especially in children (Wargo, Wargo, & Alderman, 2006). Global warming is another result of these emissions, with predictions that in the not-so-distant future it will cost millions of lives, especially in coastal areas (Perera & Sanford, 2011). And again, while the use of these fossil fuels creates profits in the short term, in the long term it will cost us billions of dollars.

There are also some government policies that harm people's health. Corn subsidies are an example. Currently in the United States, farmers are incentivized to produce corn, allowing corn and high fructose corn syrup to become low-cost sweeteners in many food products. Studies suggest that high fructose corn syrup is a contributing factor to the epidemic of obesity (Bray, Nielsen, & Popkin, 2004), placing individuals at future risk for cardiac disease, diabetes, and weight-related joint damage.

The unsustainable nature of current ways of economic thinking and planning is further demonstrated by the fact that a growing number of jobs—not only in manufacturing but also in service industries, from receptionists to middle management—are being taken over by automation and robotics (Associated Press, 2013). This irreversible trend, which will further accelerate with the development and use of artificial intelligence and nanotechnology, makes it even more urgent that we find alternatives to economic systems primarily driven by consumer spending.

Nonetheless, other than calls for environmental protection and a more equitable distribution of resources, discussions about a new economic model are still stuck in the old debate between capitalism and socialism. Accordingly, some people prescribe a return to unregulated capitalism, while others argue that socialism is the solution (Asimakopoulos, 2011; Harrington, 2011). This tired old debate distracts us from developing a new economic paradigm. It obscures the fact that neither capitalism nor socialism has prevented the massive environmental problems that today threaten our very existence. It further ignores the fact that both have helped perpetuate systems of top-down rankings. Finally, it fails to recognize that neither capitalist nor socialist theories (which came out of the early industrial 18th and 19th centuries) can help meet the unprecedented challenges posed by the technological shift to the postindustrial era.

Clearly, the world has changed radically since Adam Smith, the "father" of capitalist theory, and Karl Marx, the originator of "scientific socialism," developed their ideas. But the age of these theories is not the only problem. The deeper problem is that both theories came out of times that oriented more closely to a domination system. The "divinely ordained" rule of kings was just beginning to be challenged. Men were still supposed to be "divinely ordained" to rule over the women and children in the "castles" of their homes, and the belief that anything stereotypically associated with "men's work" was superior to anything considered "women's work" was still more securely embedded in both popular and academic thinking than it is today.

One consequence of this way of thinking was that, even though both Smith and Marx wanted to improve humanity's condition, neither gave any real value to the work of caring for people or for nature. It does not seem to have crossed Smith's or Marx's minds that keeping a clean, healthy, natural environment was of any economic importance—just as neither considered the "women's work" of keeping a clean, healthy home of any economic value. Similarly, neither man considered the work of caring for children or for people's health and well-being important in economic analyses.

Rather than recognizing environmental limitations, Smith's message was that wealth would grow endlessly thanks to the "invisible hand" of the market powered by self-interest (Smith, 1776/1937). Similarly, Marx's scientific socialism gives nearly exclusive importance to the commodification of labor, with hardly any attention to the devastating impact of industrialization on nature (Marx &

Engels, 1843-44/1960). In accordance with Marxist theory, this industrialization was then vigorously pushed in the former Soviet Union and China.

Smith and Marx considered caring for people (starting in childhood) "women's work" and as merely "reproductive" labor—not part of their "productive" economic equation. This distinction between productive and reproductive labor has been at the core of both capitalist and socialist thinking, which hardly ever considers the value of care and caregiving. This distinction persists despite its lack of accuracy, despite mounting evidence that not caring for our natural environment is potentially suicidal, and even despite findings from neuroscience that caring for people, starting in early childhood, is key to producing the "high quality human capital" economists never tire of telling us is most important for national success in the postindustrial knowledge/service economy.

Rethinking Economics

Even today, standard economics and business texts and courses fail to take into account the enormous economic value of care. This exclusion continues despite the growing number of studies showing that companies that care for employees and their families are more successful than those that do not (Eisler, 2007). For example, studies show that companies rated as the best companies to work for—companies with caring policies—have both a higher return to investors and greater customer satisfaction evaluations. To illustrate:

- Companies on the *Working Mother's* list of "100 Best Companies for Working Mothers"—companies offering more child care benefits, flexible scheduling, telecommuting, and other caring policies—had higher customer satisfaction ratings. This satisfaction translated into a 3–11% market value increase over companies without these employee-friendly policies, or $22,000 per employee (Burud &Tumulo, 2004).

- Companies rated by *Fortune* as the best places to work yielded shareholder returns on investment of 27.5%—much higher than the Russell 3000 stocks, which had average returns of 17.3% (Burud & Tumulo, 2004).

Some academics are beginning to take these kinds of findings into account. The theme of environmental sustainability is also gaining more ground. However, the economic value of caring business and government policies is still not generally part of the curriculum. And the economic value of the work of care performed in the nonmarket economy continues to be completely ignored.

Indeed, the texts assigned in most economic classes still define the domain of economics as composed only of the market, the government, and (to some extent) the illegal economic sectors (Figure 13.1). This incomplete economic map severely constrains advances toward new economic thinking.

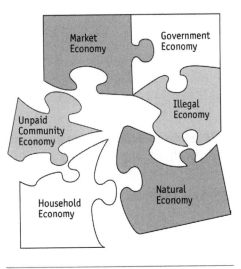

FIGURE 13.1 OLD ECONOMIC MAP.

Reprinted from Riane Eisler (2007) The Real Wealth of Nations: Creating a Caring Economy *(San Francisco, CA: Berrett-Koehler)*

As Eisler (2007) notes, when caring for people, beginning in early childhood is the starting point for economic thinking; we can move from the old economic map—the basis of both capitalist and socialist theory—to what she calls *a full-spectrum economic map* for a new, more adaptive way of thinking about and structuring economic systems (Figure 13.2).

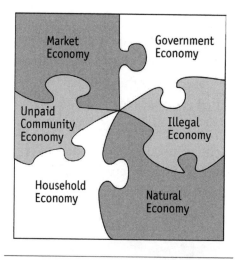

FIGURE 13.2 NEW ECONOMIC MAP.

Reprinted from Riane Eisler (2007) The Real Wealth of Nations: Creating a Caring Economy (San Francisco, CA: Berrett-Koehler)

A full-spectrum economic map includes not only the market economy, the government economy, and the illegal economy, but also the three vital *life-sustaining* economic sectors: the household economy, the natural economy, and the volunteer economy (Eisler, 2007).

This more accurate, inclusive map is an important step toward recognizing the economic importance of our natural environment and the economic value of unpaid care work—the work that sustains all of us, children, the elderly, and anyone who is sick. It is also an important step toward no longer thinking of this work as merely *reproductive work* but rather as *productive work*—an old distinction a number of scholars have noted stands in the way of a more equitable economic system (Crittenden, 2001; Eisler, 2007, 2012; Folbre, 2001; Jain & Banerjee, 1985; Kabeer, 2003; Nelson, 2006). Indeed, both leaving this antiquated distinction behind *and* embracing a full-spectrum economic map are essential if the work of care is to be given the recognition it merits. It is also a prerequisite for a new economic paradigm: one that not only promotes human survival but full human development (Eisler, 2007, 2012).

Eisler (2007) has proposed the term *partnerism* to describe what she calls *a caring economics* that goes beyond both capitalism and socialism, arguing that this is essential if we are to effectively address the unprecedented social, economic, and environmental challenges we face. However, she emphasizes that developing such a system does not mean we should discard everything from earlier theories. We need both markets and government planning.

But markets and government planning are not enough unless they give real visibility and value to the most essential human work: the work of caring for our natural environment and caring for people, starting with children, to caring for our growing aging population (Eisler, 2007).

TABLE 13.1 Comparing Standard Economics with Caring Economics

OLD ECONOMICS	PARTNERISM
Domain of economics is confined to the market, government, and illegal sectors	Domain of economics includes the life-sustaining/enhancing household, volunteer, and natural sectors
Focus on consumer spending and short-term monetary profits	Focus on long-term personal, business, and economic health
Social investment in caring for and educating people is regarded as "soft" and not of economic value	Social investment in caring for and educating people is recognized as essential for a healthy economy
Nature is here to be exploited	Nature is valued and respected
Artificial scarcity is created through war, waste, and failure to invest in human capacity development	Investment in human capacity, development, and savings from over-consumption, waste, and wars are basis for a good living standard for all
People are viewed as cogs in an economic machine	People's needs and aspirations are viewed as paramount
"Hard" stereotypically masculine values and goals such as winning over opponents are given priority by both men and women	"Soft" stereotypically feminine values such as mutual benefit and caring are given priority by both women and men
Supporting creativity is associated with the feminine role and devalued	Personal and organizational support is highly valued as the essential matrix for creativity
Care work in households is seen as "women's work" and not included in measures of economic productivity	Care work in households by both women and men is valued and included in measures of economic productivity

Some people will argue that there is no way of quantifying the value of care work. Certainly, some matters cannot be quantified, such as the enormous sense of well-being that humans feel when they receive care. However, a good deal of the economic value of the work of care can be, and already is being, quantified. Largely thanks to the activism of women's organizations worldwide, many nations have now developed "satellite" accounts that quantify the value of such work as caring for people in families and keeping healthy home environments. For example, a 2004 Swiss government report showed that if the unpaid "caring" household work still primarily performed by women were included, it would comprise 40% of the reported Swiss GDP (Schiess and Schön-Bühlmann, 2004). Unfortunately satellite accounts do not get the publicity of economic measures such as GDP. But they are a start in the right direction.

Reports by nongovernmental organizations also show the enormous value of the work of care. A recent example is *Counting on Care Work in Australia* (Hoenig & Page, 2012), a comprehensive quantification of the Australian care sector, paid and unpaid. The study used both *replacement value* (which reflects the low pay of care work in the market) and *opportunity cost* (which yields a higher value on average, measuring the lost opportunity cost for individuals who perform unpaid care instead of entering the paid work force). The study found that the care sector in Australia was worth an estimated $762.5 billion in 2009-10. Of this total, $112.4 billion was for paid care and $650.1 billion was for unpaid care work. The latter was the equivalent of no less than 50.6% of GDP. Another key finding was that women contributed the majority of this unpaid care, similar to other world regions (Hoenig, & Page, 2012).

The Australian report pointed out that care work is a "public good" and that, given its profound implications for a nation's overall well-being, government intervention in the form of public policy and funding is required to ensure that appropriate levels of care are available (Hoenig & Page, 2012).

While data showing the huge economic value of care work continue to accumulate, they are still given scant attention by academics, media, policymakers, and the public. A major reason for this neglect is that the information does not fit into the old economic paradigms or the old ways of measuring economic health such as GDP. This is why the development of new measures of economic health such as the Social Wealth Indicators being developed by the Center for Partnership Studies (CPS) discussed at the end of this chapter are so important.

Economics and Society

The problem, however, is deeper. The underlying problem is that economic systems are profoundly influenced by the larger societies in which they are embedded and by the values that people in a society believe are normal, desirable, or inevitable.

To understand the dynamic, self-organizing interaction between economics and other social institutions, as well as the impact of cultural beliefs on what is (or is not) valued, this section briefly returns to the matter we discussed in Chapter 3: the need for new ways of classifying human societies. As you saw in that chapter, conventional social categories—religious versus secular, rightist versus leftist, Eastern versus Western, or industrial versus pre- or post-industrial—cannot help us understand why caring and caregiving have been so devalued. Indeed, none of these categories describe the totality of a society's beliefs, institutions, and relationships.

This is why we use the categories of the *partnership system* and the *domination system*. These more comprehensive categories describe two very different configurations of beliefs, institutions, and relationships—from the family and education to politics and economics—as well as two very different systems of values that in turn directly affect a society's policies (Eisler, 1987a, 2002, 2007).

To briefly recap, the configuration of the *domination system* has four mutually supporting core components:

- Top-down control in *both* families and states or tribes

- Rigid male dominance and the devaluation by both men and women of anything stereotypically considered "feminine," including care and caregiving

- The acceptance and often idealization of violence as a means of imposing one's will on others

- A system of beliefs that presents relations of dominating or being dominated as inevitable and desirable

By contrast, the configuration of the *partnership system* consists of the following four mutually supporting core components:

- A more democratic and egalitarian structure in *both* the family and state or tribe

- Equal partnership between women and men, and with this, a high valuing (in women and men, as well as in social and economic policy) of traits and activities stereotypically considered "feminine," such as care and caregiving

- A low degree of abuse and violence, because they are not needed to maintain rigid rankings of domination

- A system of beliefs that presents partnership and mutual respect as normal and desirable (Eisler, 1987a, 2002, 2007)

No society orients completely to a domination system or a partnership system. It is always a matter of degree in what Eisler calls a *partnership/domination continuum*. But with these configurations in mind, much that otherwise seems random and disconnected begins to fall into place, including how economic systems have been developed.

For instance, if you look at the criticism of capitalism as unjust and exploitive, you see that in reality it is a critique not of capitalism *per se*, but of the beliefs, institutions, and relationships inherent in domination systems, whether these systems are ancient or modern, Western or Eastern, feudal, monarchic, or totalitarian (Eisler, 2007, 2012). You then see that long before capitalist billionaires amassed huge fortunes, Egyptian pharaohs and Chinese emperors hoarded their nations' wealth. Indian potentates demanded tributes of silver and gold, while lower castes lived in abject poverty. Middle Eastern warlords pillaged, plundered, and terrorized their people. European feudal lords killed their neighbors and oppressed their subjects. In all these precapitalist times and places, the gap between haves and have-nots was huge, and the mass of people had little if any chance to improve their lot. In short, all these are examples of economics in a rigid domination system.

Then look at unregulated capitalism (sometimes curiously called *neo-liberalism*) through the analytical lens of the partnership/domination continuum. You can then see that it is basically a reconsolidation of wealth and power in the hands of those on top. The rhetoric may be about freedom, but what this really means is freedom for those on top to do what they wish, free from government environmental or financial regulations (Eisler, 2012). In the same way, *trickle-down economics* is not really new. It is a return to the "traditional" order, where those on the bottom are socialized to content themselves with the crumbs dropping from their masters' opulent tables.

Not coincidentally, in domination economics (ancient or modern) you also see a marked contempt for the "soft" or stereotypically "feminine." This is exemplified by today's vitriolic attacks in the United States on the "nanny state." Again not coincidentally, this attack accompanied the current retreat from the "war on poverty" that had brought social safety nets such as Medicare for the elderly and Medicaid for people living in poverty.

Viewed from the perspective of the partnership-domination continuum, a number of other connections also become visible. You can then see that along with the current U.S. retreat from the values of the 1960s and early 1970s, when there was concern for society's most vulnerable—such as children, minorities, the poor, the disabled, and the elderly—has come the attempt to push women back into their "traditional" place through legislative and judicial restrictions on women's freedoms and opportunities. For instance, there has been a massive drive to deprive women of reproductive choice, resistance to equal pay for equal work, and even attempts to obstruct the reauthorization of the Violence against Women Act.

In other words, the push to slash government programs supporting "soft" or stereotypically feminine activities—caring for children and aid to poor families—is inextricably interconnected with the so-called "war against women." Attempts to defund Social Security, Medicare, and other social insurance programs by invoking fiscal responsibility are simply another way of taking funding from programs that care for people and instead funneling billions of dollars to big banks, powerful insurance companies, and other corporations (Eisler, 2007, 2012).

Many of the shortcomings in both capitalist and socialist theory also make more sense when you look at them through the analytical lenses of the partnership and domination systems. You can then see that Adam Smith developed capitalist theory in a time when ranking "superiors" over "inferiors" was still viewed as normal and moral, whether it was ranking kings over their "subjects," trading companies over colonized peoples, "superior" races over "inferior" ones, or men over women. In other words, capitalism was developed in a culture that was still oriented more to the domination side of the partnership/domination continuum.

Similarly, while Marx's theories came out of times when there were already organized challenges to these rankings, "scientific socialism" reflected and perpetuated domination assumptions, including the devaluation of women and anything stereotypically associated with women, such as care and caregiving (Eisler, 2007, 2012). Moreover, when Marx's goal of a "dictatorship of the proletariat" was realized in the former Soviet Union and China, it was in cultures where a rigid domination system had long been established. So, not surprisingly, authoritarianism, violence, and male dominance remained the norm.

By contrast, societies that orient more closely to the partnership side of the continuum are able to enact economic policies that combine positive elements of socialism and capitalism yet go beyond both by prioritizing care for people and nature. For example, nations such as Sweden, Finland, Norway, and Iceland lean toward the partnership configuration. These are not ideal nations, but they have more democracy and equality in both the family and the state; women have higher status (over 40% of their national legislators are female versus less than 20% in the United States); and they are in the forefront of efforts to leave behind traditions of abuse and violence. For example, these countries pioneered the first peace studies, enacted the first laws prohibiting physical discipline of children in families, and have a strong men's movement to disentangle "masculinity" from its equation with domination and violence (Eisler, 2007).

At the beginning of the 20th century, these nations were so poor that there were famines. But today they have very low poverty rates, low crime rates, and a generally high standard of living for all. A major factor in this move from poverty to prosperity is that these nations invested in caring for their people. These countries have government-supported child care, universal health care, stipends to help families care for children, elder care with dignity, and generous paid parental leave. Because they also provide good family planning and encourage women to enter the paid labor force, social support for raising children has not led to a population explosion. As a result of such policies, these nations regularly rank high in both the United Nations annual Human Development Reports measuring quality of life and the World Economic Forum's annual Global Competitiveness reports (Schwab, 2010).

Not coincidentally, these nations also take better care of the natural environment. They are ahead of most nations in meeting goals of environmental sustainability. They pioneered environmentally sound industrial approaches such as the Swedish Natural Step, where materials used to manufacture a product (from rugs to electronics) are recycled (Bradbury & Clair, 1999).

Some of the first experiments in industrial democracy also came from Sweden and Norway, as did studies showing that a more participatory structure, where workers play a part in deciding how to organize tasks and what hours to work, can be extremely effective in terms of productivity (Haug, 2004). In addition, Nordic nations have a long history of *business cooperatives*, jointly owned and democratically controlled enterprises whose concern for the surrounding community is a guiding principle.

With the globalization of unregulated capitalism, Nordic nations began moving toward more privatization. Nonetheless, they have maintained most of their caring policies and, hence, their high rankings in international surveys of quality of life (from environmental and human rights ratings to infant mortality rates). By contrast, the United States has been falling behind every industrialized nation and even some developing nations in these international rankings (Central Intelligence Agency, 2011).

A basic reason that Nordic nations rank so highly is that they continue investing resources in caring for people and nature. Indeed, these nations contribute a larger percentage of their GDP than other developed nations to caring for other nations. They also fund and provide programs working for fair economic development, environmental protection, and human rights (Organization for Economic Co-operation and Development, n.d.)

This leads to an important point. It has sometimes been said that Nordic nations have a greater investment in their human and environmental infrastructure because they are relatively small and homogeneous. Their investment in helping people from all world regions contradicts this claim. Moreover, in smaller, even more homogeneous societies (such as some oil-rich Middle-Eastern nations) where absolute conformity to one religious sect and one tribal or royal head is demanded, you find huge gaps between haves and have-nots, rigid female subordination, and a heavy reliance on fear and force to maintain their domination systems.

So clearly other factors explain why Nordic nations have a more caring, equitable economic system. One important factor, still ignored in mainstream economic analyses, is greater equality between the male and female halves of humanity. That equality is illustrated by the fact that women can, and do, occupy the highest political offices and comprise a large percentage of national legislatures. This is certainly not the only factor, but the higher status of Nordic women has had important consequences for the values that guide Nordic policies.

As explained in Chapter 3 of this book, men in domination-oriented systems are socialized to distance themselves from women and anything stereotypically considered feminine, lest they be tagged with humiliating labels such as "wimp," "sissy," or "effeminate." By contrast, in partnership-oriented cultures, men can give more value to care, caregiving, nonviolence, and other traits and activities deemed inappropriate for men in domination societies. So, along with the higher status of Nordic women, many men and women back more caring policies—policies that give value and visibility to the work of caring for people and nature (Eisler, 2007).

Economics, Values, and Gender

This correlation between the status of women and a nation's economic policies bears directly on two matters of particular importance for nursing:

- The status of the nursing profession in the new interprofessional teams now forming

- A nation's policies regarding the maintenance of its people's health and their recovery from illnesses and/or accidents

We have looked at the challenge nurses face in achieving equal status (and with this, equal voice and respect) in interprofessional teams. Here we only reiterate the point that since nursing has been primarily "women's work" and the work of care has stereotypically been considered feminine rather than masculine, the move to a partnership social configuration (and especially toward one of its key components: equal partnership between women and men) is of critical importance for advancing the nursing profession. That more men are entering nursing is a sign we are moving toward these goals, since only as the status of women rises do men feel comfortable being associated with the "feminine." Another positive sign is that more women are becoming physicians.

However, much more is needed. We must show our nation's policymakers the necessity for enacting more caring policies. There is a connection between the status of women and whether caring and caregiving are valued. Therefore, we must also show policymakers the necessity of raising the status of women worldwide.

An important tool for furthering this goal consists of empirical studies showing the connection between the status of women on the one hand and a nation's quality of life and economic success on the other. A pioneering study in this area was "Women, Men, and the Global Quality of Life," conducted by the Center for Partnership Studies (CPS) in 1995. Using data from 89 nations, it compared the status of women with measures of quality of life (such as infant mortality, human rights ratings, and environmental ratings) and showed that in significant respects, the status of women can be a better predictor of quality of life than GDP (Eisler, Loye, & Norgaard, 1995).

Since then, other studies have verified the relationship between the status of women, a society's values, and its overall quality of life and economic success. Based on data from 65 societies representing 80% of the world's population, the World Values Survey (Inglehart, Norris, & Welzel, 2002) is the largest international survey of how attitudes correlate with economic development and political structure. When for the first time this survey focused attention on attitudes about gender, it found a strong relationship between the level of support for gender equality and a society's level of political rights, civil liberties, and quality of life.

More recently, in the World Economic Forum's *Global Gender Gap Reports*, researchers Hausmann, Tyson, and Zahedi, (2011) showed that the nations with the lowest gender gaps (such as Norway, Sweden, and Finland) are also regularly in the highest ranks of the World Economic Forum's *Global Competitiveness Reports*.

Of course, the simple fact that women are half of humanity is a reason for the correlation between the status of women and national economic success and quality of life. But the reasons for this correlation go much deeper, to the still largely unrecognized interconnected cultural, social, and economic dynamics inherent in domination systems or partnership systems. In addition to the connection between a higher status of women and values and policies that support caring for people, there are a myriad other factors, including yet another matter ignored in conventional economic analyses: how resources are distributed not only within nations, but within households.

Eisler and other scholars call this *intra-household economics* (Eisler, 2007; Jain & Banerjee, 1985), and it is once again directly related to the status of women in a society. Empirical evidence across diverse cultures and income groups shows that in cultures where women are rigidly subordinated, the distribution of household resources tends to be skewed in ways that fail to invest in children's well-being, health, and development. Studies also show that in these domination-oriented cultures, women have a higher propensity than men to spend on goods that benefit children and enhance their capacities.

For example, in "Intra-Household Resource Allocation," Duncan Thomas (1990) found that $1 in the hands of a Brazilian woman had the same effect on child survival as $18 in the hands of a man. Similarly, Bruce and Lloyd (1997) found that in Guatemala an additional $11.40 per month in a mother's hands would result in the same weight gain in a young child as an additional $166 earned by the father.

Of course, even in rigidly male-dominated cultures there are men who give primary importance to meeting their families' needs. However, the socialization of men in such cultures teaches them to believe it is their prerogative to use their wages for nonfamily purposes, including drinking, smoking, and gambling (and that when women complain, they are nagging and controlling).

The negative effects of the subordination of females to males on intra-household resources distribution go even further. In some world regions, parents (both mothers and fathers) often deny girls access to education, give them less health care, and even feed girls less than boys. Obviously, these practices have terrible health consequences for girls and women. Indeed, these practices are horrendous human rights violations that not only stunt girls' development, but all too often cause their death. But giving less food to girls and women also adversely impacts the development of boys, as children of malnourished women are often born with poor health and below-par brain development (Eisler, 1987b). In short, this gender-based nutritional and health care discrimination robs all children, male and female, of their potential for optimal development. This in turn affects children's and later adults' abilities to adapt to new conditions, tolerate frustration, and avoid using violence—all of which impede solutions to chronic hunger, poverty, and armed conflict, as well as the chances for a more humane, prosperous, and peaceful world for all.

Indeed, there is no realistic way to end poverty without taking into account another gender-related matter: Women represent a disproportionate percentage of the poor worldwide. For example:

- According to some estimates, 70% of those who live in *absolute poverty*—starvation or near starvation—are female (UN Women, n.d.).

- Even in the rich United States, woman-headed families are the lowest tier of the economic hierarchy (UN Women, n.d.).

- According to the United States Census Bureau (2005), the poverty rate of women over 65 is twice that of men the same age.

This high female poverty rate is not only due to wage discrimination in the market economy; it is largely due to the fact that these women are (or were for much of their lives) either full- or part-time caregivers of children or other family members. Yet because they did this essential work without pay or later Social Security or pensions, they are condemned to an old age living in poverty.

This, however, is not inevitable. It is a matter of social policies, as shown by the low poverty rates of the nations that orient more to the partnership side of the continuum we just examined, where women and stereotypically feminine values have higher status.

We want to clarify that none of this means that economic inequities based on gender are more important than those based on class, race, or other factors. These inequities are all inherent in domination systems. And in domination systems the basic template for the division of humanity into those to be served and those that serve is a male-superior/female-inferior model of our species. This template for relations then automatically is applied to ranking one race, religion, or ethnic group over a different one.

We also want to emphasize that none of this is a matter of blaming men for our problems. Indeed, in domination systems most women, like most men, have not just been passive victims but have often been active collaborators in maintaining rankings of domination (including ranking men over women) in conformity with religious and secular teachings that such rankings are divinely or genetically ordained.

What we are dealing with are systems dynamics in which the cultural construction of the roles and relations of the female and male halves of humanity play a key role in shaping social and economic institutions and the values that guide policies and practices. And this value system plays out in the distribution of resources within households, nations, and the world, with a major factor being whether a culture or subculture orients to the partnership or domination system.

Toward a Caring Economics

In *Tomorrow's Children: A Blueprint for Partnership Education in the 21st Century*, Eisler (2000) proposes that caring for life—for self, others, and nature—should be a thread running through the educational curriculum, from preschool to graduate school. Indeed, if caring for people and nature guided government and business policies, using advanced technologies to pollute and destroy our natural habitat would be inconceivable. Also inconceivable would be the financial drain of chronic wars, corruption, and greed, and the unnecessary deaths from malnutrition and disease of millions of children, women, and men every year.

We can no longer afford the human and economic drain stemming from old economic assumptions, policies, and practices that do not support a healthy society and economy. Here are some practical steps forward:

Good Care for Children

Good care and education for children are essential if we are to have the flexible, innovative, and caring people needed for the postindustrial workforce (Cleveland & Krashinsky, 2010). Psychology and neuroscience show that whether or not these capacities develop hinges largely on the quality of care and education children receive. Indeed, neuroscience shows that the quality of care and education children receive affects nothing less than the brain's neural structures (Niehoff, 1999; Perry, 2002).

You have already seen how caring policies in Nordic nations played a major role in their move from dire poverty to economic success and a good quality of life for all. Other examples abound: the enormous financial benefits from investing in parenting education and assistance, as shown by the Healthy Babies, Healthy Children program in Canada (Ontario Ministry of Health, 2003) and investing in high-quality early childhood education, as shown by follow-up studies of the U.S. Abecedarian Project (Masse & Barnett, 2011). And as nurses know, investing in children's health not only makes economic sense but also contributes to the future sustainability of the health care system.

Good Care for Elders

As the world's elderly population grows, their care must also become a social priority. Again, women have been the main caregivers of the elderly in families, but here too they have received inadequate social and economic support. This is not only unfair to the caregivers, but to those they care for.

As nurses who care for the elderly know, older people want to care for themselves as long as possible and contribute to their families and communities. When they are no longer able to do so, they want to stay in their own homes, rather than live in an institution. Yet, ironically, in the United States, insurance and government funding primarily cover institutional placement rather than offering education and support for caregiving in homes. So here, too, the United States needs economic policies that support caregiving by family members and offer them the help of nurses and others with professional education.

Shifting Funding Priorities

Inevitably, some people will argue that there is not enough money to support caregiving in families. However, what is, or is not, funded is more a matter of priorities than of money. Once we recognize that the most important investment a nation can make is in its human infrastructure, there will be many ways of funding caring for people.

One way is to shift our funding priorities away from the massive, often unnecessary and wasteful weapons and wars characteristic of domination systems. We are not arguing for unilateral disarmament, which in a world where many nations still orient closely to the domination side of the continuum would be suicidal. We are simply pointing to the irrational funding of weapons that even the Pentagon has said are not needed, yet Congress still votes to fund (Sweigart, 2012). Consider also the horrendous waste in military procurement (for example, scandals regarding $600 toilet seats) and the disproportionate investment in huge stockpiles of nuclear and other weapons that, once again, even the military deems excessive (Phelps, 2012).

Focusing on building and maintaining personal, social, and economic health is another important way to fund care for people. Nurses know it is much more prudent to use resources for primary prevention than to wait until illnesses require complex and costly treatments. Similarly, investing in quality care of children and elders now will prevent future huge expenditures of taxpayer money on costly medical care, crime, courts, prisons, lost human potential, and environmental damage.

Taxes on financial speculation and harmful activities such as making and selling unhealthy "empty calorie" foods can also fund investment in caring for people and our natural habitat. And these investments in both our natural and human infrastructure can, and should be, amortized over a period of years, as is done for investments in material infrastructure, such as machines and buildings, rather than being simply expensed.

DEVELOPING NEW MEASURES OF ECONOMIC HEALTH

What is not visible is not factored into social policies. Therefore, the Center for Partnership Studies' Caring Economy Campaign (CEC, 2011) is working to develop and bring attention to a new way of measuring a nation's economic success and quality of life through Social Wealth Indicators.

Social wealth is defined as the attributes of a society that make it possible to create and support the development of every individual's full capacities throughout the whole human life span. Social wealth indicators identify social wealth drivers, with special focus on the value of care work and the

continues

continued

contributions of women who still perform most of this work in both the market and non-market economic sectors. (Of course, we want all unpaid work time to be valued no matter which gender provides it, since more men are staying home to care for children and elders.)

Other drivers for social wealth include factors such as health care, early childhood education, and life-long education—areas with which nursing and nursing research are intimately familiar.

As a first step toward developing Social Wealth Indicators as more accurate and inclusive economic measures, the Center for Partnership Studies (CPS, n.d.) commissioned an analysis by the Urban Institute of new indicators currently being developed as alternatives and/or supplements to GDP. As reported in The State of Society: Measuring Economic Success and Human Well-Being *(de Leon & Boris, 2010), this survey found that while all these new efforts are important, the vast majority still pay scant if any attention to the economic value of the work of care, and thus also to the contributions of women who do most of this work in both the market (where it is generally low paid) and in families and communities (where it is unpaid).*

As a follow-up to this report, in 2012 the Center for Partnership Studies and the Urban Institute convened a 2-day meeting in Washington, DC, to pave the way for the development of Social Wealth Indicators. Twenty economists (including experts on the value of care work in both the paid and unpaid economic sectors and scholars specializing in the return on investment from high-quality early childhood education) discussed the development of Social Wealth Indicators and their inclusion in the new U.S. Key National Indicators System authorized by Congress, as well as in other national accounts. The proceedings and recommendations of the experts at this meeting are summarized in National Indicators and Social Wealth *(de Leon, 2012). The report outlines steps toward the gathering and development of a transdisciplinary set of social wealth indicators to more accurately measure human well-being and economic success as the basis for government and business policies.*

Currently, CPS's Caring Economy Campaign (www.caringeconomy.org) is planning further research and a Social Wealth website that will be a clearinghouse for Social Wealth Indicators as these are gathered and developed worldwide.

TWO SOCIAL WEALTH INDICATORS SUBDOMAINS

1. **Human capacity indicators** *measure the degree of human capacity development. These include existing health indicators, such as measures of maternal and infant health, life expectancy, morbidity, and mortality. They also include other health-related indicators that should be considered, such as the availability of contraception and prenatal care. Time-use surveys, showing the time women and men spend in care work, are also important. Under the category of education, indicators such as early childhood education and parenting education are particularly important.*

2. **Care investment indicators** *measure a country's national investment (from government, business, and civil society) in caring for people through both the paid and unpaid sectors. This investment is required to meet individual needs and the need for the high-quality human capital for a nation to compete and succeed in the knowledge/service-based economy.*

Conclusion

We can no longer tolerate chronic hunger and poverty, the widening gap between haves and have-nots, indiscriminate and wasteful overconsumption, and the devastation of our natural environment. We must invest in caring for people rather than killing people, and not only because it is the right thing to do, but because it is the economically sound thing to do.

By increasing government investment in childcare, health, and education, we pave the way for a future where all children have the opportunity to realize their potentials for consciousness, empathy, caring, and creativity—the capacities that make us fully human. But this will happen only if we change not only our economic theories but the policies and practices that stem from them.

This is why it is important for nursing education—and all education—to not only reexamine current economic thinking but also, as we have briefly done in this chapter, lay out tangible steps we can take to build foundations for a more humane and effective caring economy.

AN INVITATION TO NURSES FROM RIANE EISLER (POTTER, 2010)

I want to invite nurses and nurse educators to join our Center for Partnership Studies' Caring Economy Campaign (please see www.caringeconomy.org). The Caring Economy Campaign has four goals:

- *Change popular language and thinking by changing the conversation (and consciousness) to recognize the enormous value of the work of caring and caregiving, and hence the need for moving to a caring economics*

- *Empower leaders, grassroots organizations, and individuals through online information and tools, public policy alternatives, and interactive learning webinars such as the Caring Economics Leadership Programs (CELP)*

- *Inform and engage the media, both alternative and mainstream*

- *Inspire the development of new economic indicators, practices, and policies that give visibility and real value to the most important human work: the work of caring for nature and all people, starting with young children*

Nursing is, above all, a caring profession. The nursing profession has a big stake in this campaign. Nursing organizations can play a key role in the Center's work to change economic indicators to give more visibility to the enormous value of caring and caregiving. Nursing schools and organizations can also take advantage of the Caring Economy Leadership Program and Riane Eisler's Cultural Transformation Course offered online (http://www.caringeconomy.org/content/caring-economy-leadership-program). You can incorporate some of these materials into the new story of nursing.

Indeed, it is through education not only of nurses, but also of policymakers and the public at large, that the story and realities of the nursing profession can be changed in ways that will benefit us all (R. Eisler, personal communication, August 25, 2010, printed with permission).

References

Asimakopoulos, J. (2011). *Revolt! The next great transformation from kleptocracy capitalism to libertarian socialism through counter ideology, societal education, and direct action.* Fair Lawn, NJ: Transformative Studies Institute.

Associated Press (January 1, 2013) Recession, technology kill middle-class jobs. Chicago: Daily Herald. http://www.dailyherald.com/article/20130123/business/701239938/

Bradbury, H., & Clair, J. A. (1999). Promoting sustainable organizations with Sweden's natural step. *The Academy of Management Executive, 13*(4), 63-74.

Bray, G. A., Nielsen, S. J., & Popkin, B. M. (2004). Consumption of high-fructose corn syrup in beverages may play a role in the epidemic of obesity. *American Journal of Clinical Nutrition, 79*(4), 537-543.

Bruce, J., & Lloyd, C. B. (1997). Finding the ties that bind: Beyond headship and household. In L. Haddad, J. Hoddinott, & H. Alderman (Eds.), *Intra-household resources allocation in developing countries: Methods, models, and policy*. Baltimore, MD: International Food Policy Research Institute and The Johns Hopkins University Press.

Burud, S., & Tumolo, M. (2004). *Leveraging the new human capital: Adaptive strategies, results achieved, and stories of transformation*. Mountain View, CA: Davies-Black Publishing.

Caring Economy Campaign. (2011). Three reasons why we need a caring economy. Retrieved from http://www.caringeconomy.org/content/three-reasons-why-we-need-caring-economy

Center for Partnership Studies (CPS). (n.d.). CPS-commissioned urban institute report released on June 2. Retrieved from http://www.partnershipway.org/news-media-room/partnership-news/featured-news/milestone-on-road-to-caring-economics-revealed-on-june-2-2010/?searchterm=Urban%20Institute

Central Intelligence Agency (CIA). (2011). *The world factbook, country comparison: Infant mortality rates, 2011*. Retrieved from https://www.cia.gov/library/publications/the-world-factbook/rankorder/2091rank.html

Cleveland, G., & Krashinsky, M. (2010). The benefits and costs of good childcare: The economic rationale for public investment in young children—A policy study. In P. Kershaw, & L. Anderson (Eds.), *Smart Family Policies for Strong Economies*. Retrieved from http://www.learn-council.ca/FamilyLiteracy_3_1580827437.pdf

Crittenden, A. (2001). *The price of motherhood: Why the most important job in the world is still the least valued*. New York, NY: Metropolitan Books.

de Leon, E. (2012). *National indicators and social wealth*. Washington, DC: The Urban Institute.

de Leon, E., & Boris, E.T. (2010). *The state of society: Measuring economic success and human well-being.* Washington, DC: The Urban Institute.

Eisler, R. (1987a). *The chalice and the blade: Our history, our future.* San Francisco, CA: HarperCollins.

Eisler, R. (1987b). Human rights: Toward an integrated theory for action. *The Human Rights Quarterly, 9*(3), 287-308.

Eisler, R. (2000). *Tomorrow's children: A blueprint for partnership education in the 21ˢᵗ century.* Boulder, CO: Westview Press.

Eisler, R. (2002). *The power of partnership: Seven relationships that will change your life.* Novato, CA: New World Publishing.

Eisler, R. (2007). *The real wealth of nations: Creating a caring economics.* San Francisco, CA: Berret-Koehler.

Eisler, R. (2012). Economics as if caring matters. *Challenge, 55*(2), 58-86.

Eisler, R., Loye, D., & Norgaard, K. (1995). *Women, men, and the global quality of life.* Pacific Grove, CA: Center for Partnership Studies.

Folbre, N. (2001). *The invisible heart: Economics and family values.* New York, NY: New Press.

Harrington, M. (2011). *Socialism: Past and future.* New York, NY: Arcade Publishing.

Haug, R. (2004). The history of industrial democracy in Sweden: Industrial revolution to 1980. *International Journal of Management, 21*(1).

Hausmann, R., Tyson, L. D., & Zahidi, S. S. (2011). *The global gender gap report.* Geneva, Switzerland: The World Economic Forum.

Hoenig, S. A., & Page, A. R. E. (2012). *Counting on care work in Australia.* Australia: AEC*group* Limited economic Security4Women (eS4W). Retrieved from http://www.security4women.org.au/wp-content/uploads/eS4W-Counting-on-Care-Work-in-Australia-Final-Report.pdf

Inglehart, R., Norris, P., & Welzel, C. (2002). Gender equality and democracy. *Comparative Sociology, 1*(3-4), 321-346.

Investopedia. (2013). Gross domestic product—GDP. Retrieved from http://www.investopedia.com/terms/g/gdp.asp

Jain, D., & Banerjee, N. (1985). *The tyranny of the household: Women and poverty.* New Delhi, India: Shakti Books.

Kabeer, N. (2003). *Gender mainstreaming in poverty eradication and the millennium development goals: A handbook for policy-makers and other stakeholders.* Commonwealth Secretariat/IDRC/CIDA.

Marx, K., & Engels, F. (1960). *Werke, 8.* Berlin: Dietz Verlag. (Original work published 1843-44)

Masse, L. N., & Barnett, W. S. (2011). *A benefit cost analysis of the Abecedarian early childhood intervention.* New Brunswick, NJ: National Institute for Early Education Research, Rutgers, State University of New Jersey.

Nelson, J. (2006). *Economics for humans.* Chicago, IL: University of Chicago Press.

Niehoff, D. (1999). *The biology of violence: How understanding the brain, behavior, and environment can break the vicious circle of aggression.* New York, NY: Free Press.

Ontario Ministry of Health and Long-Term Care. (2003). Healthy babies healthy children report card. Retrieved from www.health.gov.on.ca/english/public/pub/ministry_reports/healthy_babies_report/hbabies_report.html

Organization for Economic Co-operation and Development (OECD). (n.d.). Development aid rose in 2009 and most donors will meet 2010 aid targets. Retrieved from http://www.oecd.org/investment/stats/developmentaidrosein2009andmostdonorswillmeet2010aidtargets.htm

Perera, E. M., & Sanford, T. (2011). Climate change and your health. Washington, DC: Union of Concerned Scientists Climate Change Program.

Perry, B. (2002). Childhood experience and the expression of genetic potential. *Brain and Mind, 3*(1), 79-100.

Phelps, M. (2012). 5 weapons the Pentagon opposed but Congress approved. Retrieved from http://www.listosaur.com/politics/5-weapons-the-pentagon-opposed-but-congress-approved.html

Potter, T. M. (2010). Reconstructing a new story of nursing: Critical analysis of nursing textbooks using Riane Eisler's partnership paradigm. *Dissertation Abstracts International, 72*(05), 3447086.

Schiess, U., & Schön-Bühlmann, J. (2004). *Satellitenkonto Haushaltsproduktion Pilotversuch für die Schweiz.* Neuchâtel, Switzerland: Statistik der Schweiz.

Schram, C. (2011). Is the financial sector gobbling up the U.S.' would-be entrepreneurs? *Forbes.* April 13. Retrieved from http://www.forbes.com/2011/04/12/financial-sector-mba-entrepreneurs-opinions-contributors-carl-schramm_2.html

Schwab, K. (Ed.). (2010). *The global competitiveness report 2010-2011*. Geneva, Switzerland: World Economic Forum.

Smith, A. (1937). *The wealth of nations*. New York: Modern Library. (Original work published in 1776).

Stewart, H. (2010, September 19). Consumer spending and the economy. *New York Times*. Retrieved from http://fivethirtyeight.blogs.nytimes.com/2010/09/19/consumer-spending-and-the-economy/

Sweigart, J. (2012, August 20). Congress pushes for weapons Pentagon didn't want. *Dayton Daily News*. Retrieved from http://www.military.com/daily-news/2012/08/20/congress-pushes-for-weapons-pentagon-didnt-want.html

Thomas, D. (1990). Intra-household resource allocation: An inferential approach. *Journal of Human Resources, 25*(4), 635-664.

UN Women. (n.d.). *Women, poverty, and economics*. Retrieved from http://www.unifem.org/gender_issues/women_poverty_economics/

United Nations Development Programme. (2013). Human development report 2011. New York, NY. Retrieved from http://hdr.undp.org/en/reports/global/hdr2011/

United States Census Bureau. (2005). Appendix: Selected highlights from 65+ in the United States: 2005. Retrieved from http://www.census.gov/newsroom/releases/archives/news_conferences/2006-03-09_appendix.html

Wargo, J., Wargo, L., & Alderman, N. (2006). *The harmful effects of vehicle exhaust: A case for policy change*. North Haven, CT: Environment & Human Health, Inc.

Chapter 14
Leading the Change

"Where after all do universal human rights begin? In small places, closest to home—so close and so small that they cannot be seen on any map of the world. Yet they are the world of the individual person: The neighborhood [s]he lives in; the school or college [s]he attends; the factory, farm or office where [s]he works. Such are the places where every man, woman, and child seeks equal justice, equal opportunity, equal dignity without discrimination. Unless these rights have meaning there, they have little meaning anywhere. Without concerted citizen action to uphold them close to home, we shall look in vain for progress in the larger world."

–Eleanor Roosevelt (1958)

All around us, old institutions, including our health care systems, are in a state of flux. In the words of Kurt Lewin (1947), the founder of social psychology, it is a time of "unfreezing." As Lewin also noted, the "freezing" that follows such a time can either be another version of the old system or a new system that better meets human needs.

Throughout this book you have been on a journey toward partnership. This is the end of the book, but it is only the beginning of a new chapter in health care. The real story of nursing and health care partnerships will be played out in your own professional life, and how it plays out will be profoundly influenced by the decisions you make and the role you play in moving health care—and society at large—toward the partnership model. This book describes some actions you can take to support the work of partnership if you are a health care educator or provide direct patient or community care. But others of you in the health care profession also have important roles to play in bringing a partnership-based health care system to life.

Executive Leaders

Nursing and other health executives can play a significant role in shifting their organization toward partnership and away from domination by committing themselves to the following objectives.

Championing Hierarchies of Actualization Throughout the Organization

As you saw, hierarchies of domination limit employee engagement, adversely impact quality and safety, and hinder innovation. Executives can prevent these negative outcomes by committing themselves to building and supporting hierarchies of actualization throughout the organization.

In *The Power of Partnership*, *The Real Wealth of Nations*, and other works, Eisler (2002, 2007, 2013) describes the many benefits to organizations when hierarchies of actualization, in which everyone's contribution is valued, are the norm. In health care, these benefits manifest themselves as follows:

- **Engagement increases when employees feel valued and empowered.** Employees are more likely to participate in teams to address organization-wide challenges and implement new health care initiatives.

- **When conflicts arise, employees work together creatively to explore alternatives.** Health care in the United States is in a state of change, and conflicting opinions and approaches are common. Instead of conflict being seen as win-lose situations, employees see conflicts as opportunities to explore and cocreate better solutions.

- **Employees who feel safe and empowered are more creative at problem solving because they feel a decreased fear of punishment for risk-taking.** Hierarchies of actualization also promote the practice autonomy of nurses, which is a criterion for Magnet recognition (American Nurses Credentialing Center [ANCC], 2013, Forces of Magnetism).

- **Communication flows freely in all directions. Hierarchies of actualization promote personal safety, which is reflected in increased patient safety.** Employees know they can report adverse working conditions and situations that negatively impact patient outcomes without fear of losing their employment. These communications lead to earlier and more effective responses. Hierarchies of actualization also promote appropriate interprofessional communication, further enhancing patient- and family-centered care.

- **Synergistic belonging extends to society and the planet, creating the social and environmental consciousness needed for long-range planning, sustainability, and success.** Hierarchies of actualization encourage employees to work together to find solutions for our most challenging health care problems, including addressing the social and economic determinants of health, environmental degradation, and climate change.

Providing and Championing Family-Friendly Policies and Practices

Employers can see additional benefits when other partnership-based policies are put in place:

- **When the workplace is family-friendly, benefits flow to employers, employees, and patients.** Family-friendly policies are essential for nurses and other health care providers who are either parents or caregivers for other relatives, including the growing elderly population. Childcare, flexible work hours, and paid sick and family leaves prevent enormous stress and promote better performance. They decrease absenteeism and attrition, with great savings on replacement and retraining costs (Burud & Tumolo, 2004; Eisler, 2007). When employees feel personally connected to the mission and vision of the organization, there is a greater sense of community and higher morale. And of course, less tense, more satisfied employees positively impact patient satisfaction scores.

- **Family-friendly policies position the hospital to be a powerful role model in the community.** Hospitals, clinics, and other health care organizations can demonstrate their partnership commitment by providing childcare, flexible work hours, and paid family leaves. Family-friendly policies also project a positive image of the organization, which has a huge marketing value.

- **By championing family-friendly policies, health care organizations can play a positive role in social policy.** As you saw in Chapter 13, the benefits of caring public policies to a nation's economic system are enormous. By advocating for family-friendly social policies at the local, national, and international levels, executives can make the case for the value of caring to both individual health and a healthy society and help show the cost-effectiveness of these investments.

Fostering Environments that Promote Partnership-Based Interprofessional Practice

Health care executives can use their power and influence to positively impact interprofessional practice. For example, leaders can review and, where necessary, change organization policies and procedures to make certain that interprofessional teamwork is supported.

Health care executives can work with nursing to ensure the organization has a zero-tolerance policy for abusive language and behavior. For a partnership system to be sustainable, existing elements of domination must be identified and transformed. No matter what the source, abuses should be quickly explored so that the dignity and safety of patients, families, and employees is protected. By providing a rapid response to reports of domination and incivility, leaders role model partnership in action.

Ensuring Implementation of Partnership Principles at Every Level of the Organization

Health care executives can strengthen the organization's commitment to partnership by creating *partnership councils* that include representation from all the units or specialties and service groups. Responsibilities of the council members include the following:

- Providing and receiving information related to effective application of the partnership model.

- Making certain that threads of domination, including episodes of abuse, are recognized and addressed with expediency.

- Cocreating new initiatives to further partnership-based health care.

The work of bringing a partnership model forward in an organization is, of course, everyone's business. But the ease of transformation from domination to partnership will be directly related to whether or not the executive leaders are committed to partnership.

HEALTH CARE EXECUTIVE LEADING THE CHANGE

"When health is absent, wisdom cannot reveal itself, art cannot become manifest, strength cannot fight, wealth becomes useless, and intelligence cannot be applied."

–Herophilus of Chalcedone, 335-280 BCE,
Physician to Alexander the Great

This ancient healing wisdom painted on the wall of Boynton Health Service, a full-service primary care clinic serving the University of Minnesota community, is a wonderful reminder of Boynton's mission to "[a]ssure students, staff, and faculty members a healthy environment in which to live and work" (University of Minnesota, 2013a, "Boynton Health Service, About Boynton Health Service").

continues

continued

To this end Director and Chief Health Officer Ferdinand Schlapper exemplifies leading with a partnership approach. He encourages each of the 300 employees of the health center to recognize the importance of their contribution to the goals and visions of the clinic. He empowers interprofessional and interdisciplinary teams to solve the most challenging health care issues. He also intentionally creates a culture where two-way communication is appreciated and encouraged; for example, leaders receive regular feedback from followers about their effectiveness as leaders.

Respect and commitment to teamwork is also extended to students. Schlapper stated, "We're going to change the world! Everyone will look to the University of Minnesota as we develop and transform today's students into tomorrow's leaders, inspiring them to discover and fulfill their life's promise and potential" (University of Minnesota, 2013b, "Strengths at the U"). That is hierarchy of actualization at work!

Professional Nursing Organizations

Frontline care providers cannot shift the health care system toward partnership without support from external stakeholders, especially leaders of nursing organizations such as the American Nurses Association (ANA), the International Council of Nurses (ICN), Sigma Theta Tau International (STTI), and the National Council of State Boards of Nursing (NCSBN). All these professional organizations influence the direction of health care by:

- Providing best practice guidelines for their members

- Supporting ongoing nursing scholarship

- Advocating for local, national, and international policies that support nursing practice, education, and research

But these organizations also play a major role in leading members to advocate for the better health of communities through both personal life changes and more caring business and social policies.

Furthermore, the NCSBN is responsible for the development of the national nursing licensure exams. This responsibility offers a tremendous opportunity to further the paradigm shift toward partnership. For example, leaders at the NCSBN can ensure that partnership competencies such as interprofessional practice and patient- and family-centered care are included in the exam. There is a powerful connection between the exam plan and nursing education curricula. In addition, nursing education organizations such as the American Association of Colleges of Nursing (AACN) and the National League for Nursing (NLN) also need to become involved. These organizations link education and practice and are therefore well-positioned to address the severe interprofessional education and practice gap.

As you have seen, health care is both influenced by, and in turn influences, the larger social and economic system. This is why health care leaders must engage in forward-looking dialogues with leaders in the fields of insurance, food production, and other businesses whose products directly impact the health of communities, as well as with policymakers on the local, national, and international levels.

In sum, leaders of professional organizations can significantly promote the partnership model by working to embrace and promote principles of partnership in both their organizations and society at large. Nurse advocates can also use Eisler's *cultural transformation theory* (1987, 2002) and *caring economics theory* (2007) to ensure that local, federal, and international governments support partnership. Another excellent resource is Riane Eisler's Cultural Transformation Course (www.caringeconomy.org).

Eisler (2002, 2007, 2013) describes many actions that we can take in the political arena to foster a shift toward partnership:

- Promote the election of local, national, and international leaders who promote democracy, equality, respect, and dignity for all, especially those without traditional access to power.

- Challenge popular media when it promotes unhealthy lifestyles.

- Encourage our political representatives to promote legislation that:

  - Ends child poverty

  - Promotes partnership education in schools

  - Funds high-quality childcare

  - Funds family-friendly policies such as paid sick leave, paid parental leave, and other measures vital for a healthier and less stressed population

  - Prevents violence against women, which the World Health Organization (WHO, 2013) has identified as one of the most serious health problems in the world today

  - Prevents and prosecutes violence against children of both genders as well as against the elderly, which are also major international health problems (Eisler, 2013)

  - Increases gender balance and female leadership and encourages participation of diverse communities in government

  - Ensures adequate education, status, and economic rewards for those who perform the essential work of caring in our homes and communities

  - Supports socially and environmentally responsible business standards and rules

  - Supports a whole systems approach to health care, including adequate nutrition, economic security, quality education, and protection of our natural environment

The knowledge and views of health care professionals are deeply respected by health care consumers and many politicians. It is therefore critical for health care leaders to continue promoting and modeling active involvement in shifting local, national, and international policy toward partnership.

AN ORGANIZATION LEADING THE CHANGE

Foundations also play a key role in leading the change. In health care, the Robert Wood Johnson Foundation (RWJF) exemplifies partnership values. The mission statement of the RWJF includes, "We harness the power of partnerships by bringing together key players, collaborating with colleagues, and securing the sustained commitment of other funders and advocates to improve the health and health care of all Americans" (RWJF, n.d., "Our Mission")

During its 40-year history the RWJF has consistently played a significant role in promoting change at a systems level. Often their success lies in their willingness to challenge traditional hierarchies of domination. In their report From the Bottom Up, the RWJF (2012) detailed the partnership-based process that has yielded such significant outcomes.

"[W]e:

- *Listened to the small voices of our most at-risk, isolated and vulnerable people.*
- *Gave stature and standing to a small and fragmented field.*
- *Created a public-private alliance of partners.*
- *Designed a way to meet the needs of disabled and elderly Americans.*
- *Put the design to the test in small pieces.*
- *Measured, evaluated and measured again.*
- *Tested, perfected and replicated the model.*
- *Attracted support among state and federal policy-makers.*
- *Used change on an intimate, personal level to leverage system change." (p. 5)*

In all of its actions, the RWJF is clearly leading the change.

Research

The field of interprofessional practice is still relatively young, so many important areas of research are yet to be explored. We particularly encourage researchers to explore the following questions related to partnership:

- What is the impact on patient outcomes when patients and families experience full implementation of patient- and family-centered care?

- What impact do poverty and other aspects of domination systems have on health?

- How does the gendered system of values that marginalizes women and the stereotypically "feminine," such as caring, caregiving, and nonviolence, affect funding of health care?

- How do cultural traditions that do not permit women to seek health or reproductive care without male permission affect access to health care?

- How do traditions of violence against women and children adversely affect health?

- How does a diverse health care workforce impact prevention and healing?

- How can the format of electronic health records support the full partnership of patients?

- How can the format of electronic health records support partnership-based interprofessional practice?

- What are the practice outcomes when nurses are educated in the full BASE of Nursing (Potter, 2013), described in Chapter 1?

- What lessons can be learned from the lived experience of earlier health care leaders?

- Which actions support the healing potential of nature?

- Which education experiences best prepare students to be effective members of interprofessional practice teams?

- What difference does health care professional self-care have on patient satisfaction?

- How can nurses most effectively prevent intra-nursing incivility and bullying?

- How can research best promote and respond to community-driven health-related questions?

- What impact do caring economic policies have on the Triple Aim, described in Chapter 2?

These questions barely scratch the surface. We must continue to drive the creation of knowledge that demonstrates both the harm of domination and the health benefits of partnership. We encourage nurse researchers and scholars in related fields to use principles of partnership and caring economics to guide your inquiries, determine your participant groups, and influence dissemination of your findings. Your contribution to the knowledge of partnership is a critical aspect of shifting the paradigm.

RESEARCH LEADING THE CHANGE

Metrics can be a powerful impetus for change. For instance:

- **Infant mortality rates:** *According to the 2013 CIA World Fact Book, the United States ranks 174th of 224 nations, with every industrialized nation and poorer nations such as Andorra, Malta, and Cuba having fewer infant deaths per 1,000 live births (Central Intelligence Agency [CIA], 2013)*

- **Maternal mortality rates:** *The United States ranks 137th out of 184 countries, behind poorer nations and countries with significant social challenges, such as the Balkans (CIA, 2013).*

- **Health care costs:** *The United States spends much more on health care than any other industrialized country. The United States spends 17.9% of its gross domestic product (GDP) on health care, more than 189 other nations (CIA, 2013).*

- **Health care delivery recipient satisfaction:** *According to the 2008 Commonwealth Fund survey, compared to six other developed nations, the United States ranks last or next to last on quality, access, efficiency, equity, and healthy lives (Davis, Schoen, & Stremikis, 2010).*

Referring to these statistics, the Caring Economy Campaign concludes with this call to action: "These are sobering statistics that must be brought to the attention of policymakers and the American public. They demonstrate the urgent need for reassessing U.S. government policies and business practices" (Caring Economy Campaign, n.d.).

Global Challenges for Interprofessional Teams

Many of the most critical health-justice issues are directly related to systems of domination. Partnership-based interprofessional teams are necessary to solve challenging global health issues such as:

- Female genital mutilation, continued lack of access to adequate family planning, denial of access to maternal health care, selective female infanticide, sexual abuse of women and children, denial to girl children of food and health care, sex trafficking, and the worldwide epidemic of violence against women and children (Eisler, 2013)

- Health disparities related to poverty, inequalities in access to health care and health education, and the burden of environmentally related illnesses that disproportionately impact poor communities (Centers for Disease Control and Prevention [CDC], n.d.)

- The disproportionate burden of disease such as tuberculosis, hepatitis, HIV/AIDS in developing nations (Prüss-Üstün & Corvalán, 2006)

- Neglected tropical diseases (NTDs): illnesses that disproportionately affect developing nations and the poor so research and development into new treatment options are limited (Hotez, 2013)

These are just a few of the global health challenges that stem from the failure to apply partnership-based principles. Indeed, dismantling domination systems with partnership approaches is the only way to see progress on these issues that threaten millions of lives.

GLOBAL NONPROFIT LEADING THE CHANGE

The nonprofit organization Unite for Sight uses interprofessional teams to address a significant global health care disparity. Unite for Sight provides financial and human resources to meet the eye care needs of the world's most impoverished communities. Much of their success lies in their work with local teams of providers and their commitment to innovation and social entrepreneurship.

In addition to providing global health care, each year Unite for Sight sponsors the world's largest global health and social entrepreneurship conference.

> *"The Global Health & Innovation Conference annually convenes more than 2,200 participants from all 50 states and more than 55 countries. The conference participants bring experience from a wide variety of disciplines, and include students, nurses, doctors, policy-makers, nonprofit directors and volunteers, public health professionals, health educators, community health workers, researchers, social scientists, social workers, social entrepreneurs, philanthropists, teachers, lawyers, and business executives. The goal of the conference is to exchange ideas and best practices across disciplines in order to improve public health and international development. Participants are encouraged to attend presentations in fields that may be outside of their existing expertise so that they can learn about successful strategies in other fields that may be applicable to their own work." (Unite for Sight, n.d., "About Us")*

The conference embodies partnership values, including respect for other professions, interprofessional collaboration to find solutions to health care challenges, and dismantling of rigid silos between specialties. The Unite for Sight Global Health and Innovation conference can serve as a model for future interprofessional conferences.

Conclusion

Chapter 13 details some of the enormous benefits from a more partnership-oriented economic system. We want to conclude this book by emphasizing this point: Partnership systems are more effective not only in human and environmental terms, but also in purely financial terms.

Indeed, partnership approaches work better in just about every sphere and every kind of relationship. For example, an illustration of the efficacy of partnership principles that Eisler (2002) cites is the success of the famous "horse whisperer" Monty Roberts. Going against the usual fear-and-force practice, Roberts applied principles of partnership by choosing to "gentle" rather than "break" young horses—with astounding results all around. Health care professionals can also choose to "gentle" rather than "break" the various relationships in health care. Instead of engaging in or condoning verbal or physical actions that limit, threaten, or control patients, colleagues, or other professionals, we can choose partnership—and together cocreate effective, sustainable, and environmentally healthy practices.

Just as Roberts' partnership approach resulted in his horses winning races all over the world, health care professionals can use the partnership approach to successfully bring quality care to individuals and communities around the globe.

We want to invite you to be part of this new era, where we all work together to cocreate a partnership-based health care system that works for everyone. As we move toward the partnership model, we can better care for others and ourselves, and—together—lay solid foundations for a healthier and more caring world.

References

American Nurses Credentialing Center (ANCC). (2013). Forces of magnetism. Retrieved from http://www.nursecredentialing.org/Magnet/ProgramOverview/HistoryoftheMagnetProgram/ForcesofMagnetism

Burud, S. & Tumolo, M. (2004). *Leveraging the new human capital: Adaptive strategies, results achieved, and stories of transformation.* Mountain View, CA: Davies-Black Publishing.

Caring Economy Campaign. (n.d.). The real wealth of nations public policy initiative: Sample fact sheet on the United States. Retrieved from http://www.caringeconomy.org/sites/default/files/imce/pdfs/912RWNUSFactsheet.pdf

Centers for Disease Control and Prevention (CDC). (n.d.). Health disparities. Retrieved from http://www.cdc.gov/healthyyouth/disparities/

Central Intelligence Agency (CIA). (2013). *The world factbook.* Retrieved from https://www.cia.gov/library/publications/the-world-factbook/rankorder/2091rank.html

Davis, K., Schoen, C., & Stremikis, K. (2010). Mirror, mirror on the wall: How the performance of the U.S. health care system performs internationally. Retrieved from http://www.commonwealthfund.org/~/media/Files/Publications/Fund%20 Report/2010/Jun/1400_Davis_Mirror_Mirror_on_the_wall_2010.pdf

Eisler, R. (1987). *The chalice and the blade: Our history, our future.* San Francisco, CA: HarperCollins.

Eisler, R. (2002). *The power of partnership: Seven relationships that will change your life.* Novato, CA: New World Library.

Eisler, R. (2007). *The real wealth of nations: Creating a caring economics.* San Francisco, CA: Berret-Koehler.

Eisler, R. (2013). Protecting the majority of humanity: Toward an integrated approach to crimes against present and future generations. In S. Jodoin & M. C. Cordonier Segger (Eds.), *Sustainable development, international criminal justice, and treaty implementation.* Cambridge, UK: Cambridge University Press.

Hotez, P. J. (2013). Addressing the neglected diseases treatment gap. Testimony before the Subcommittee on Africa, Global Health, Global Human Rights, and International Organizations, Committee on Foreign Affairs, United States House of Representatives, 113th Congress, June 27, 2013. Retrieved from http://www.sabin. org/sites/sabin.org/files/PeterJHotez%20Testimony%20Before%20House%20%20 Subcommittee%20on%20Africa%20Global%20Health%20Global%20Human%20 Rights%206%2027%202013.pdf

Lewin, K. (1947). Frontiers in group dynamics: Concept, method and reality in social science; social equilibria and social change. *Human Relations, 1,* 5-41. doi: 10.1177/001872674700100103

Potter, T. M. (2013). *The BASE of nursing.* Unpublished manuscript, School of Nursing, University of Minnesota, United States of America.

Prüss-Üstün, A. & Corvalán, C. (2006). *Preventing disease through healthy environments: Towards an estimate of the environmental burden of disease.* Geneva, Switzerland: World Health Organization.

Robert Wood Johnson Foundation (RWJF). (n.d.). Our mission. Retrieved from http:// www.rwjf.org/en/about-rwjf/our-mission.html

Robert Wood Johnson Foundation (RWJF). (2012). From the bottom up. Retrieved from http://www.rwjf.org/en/research-publications/find-rwjf-research/2012/05/from-the-bottom-up.html

Roosevelt, E. (1958). *Remarks at the United Nations, March 27, 1958.* Washington, DC: The Eleanor Roosevelt Papers Project at George Washington University. Retrieved from http://www.gwu.edu/~erpapers/abouteleanor/er-quotes/

Unite for Sight. (n.d.). Global health and innovation conference. Retrieved from http://www.uniteforsight.org/about-us

University of Minnesota. (2013a). Boynton Health Service, About Boyton Health Service. Retrieved from http://www.bhs.umn.edu/about/index.htm

University of Minnesota. (2013b). Strengths at the U. Retrieved from http://www.strengths.umn.edu/create-content/34-34/34-34-strengths-action/34-34-strengths-action-3

World Health Organization (WHO). (2013). *Global and regional estimates of violence against women: Prevalence and health effects of intimate partner violence and non-partner sexual violence.* Geneva, Switzerland: WHO Document Production Services. Retrieved from http://apps.who.int/iris/bitstream/10665/85239/1/9789241564625_eng.pdf

Index